Intr...

Den...

The Essential Facts .

D1347629

David S...

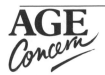

AGE *Concern*

BOOKS

©2001 David Sutcliffe

Published by Age Concern England
1268 London Road
London SW16 4ER

First published 2001

Editor Ro Lyon
Production Vinnette Marshall
Design and typesetting GreenGate Publishing Services, Tonbridge, Kent
Printed and bound in Great Britain by Bell & Bain Ltd, Glasgow

A catalogue record for this book is available from the British Library.

ISBN 0-86242-283-3

Bulk orders
Age Concern England is pleased to offer customised editions of all its titles to UK companies, institutions or other organisations wishing to make a bulk purchase. For further information, please contact the Publishing Department at the address on this page. Tel: 020 8765 7200. Fax: 020 8765 7211. Email: books@ace.org.uk

Contents

About the author

Getting a job with the Alzheimer's Society in 1984 led David Sutcliffe on a rapid learning curve as he had no previous experience of dementia. He set off on the task of developing the Society in London boroughs such as Greenwich and Bexley. He then spent time training people who were starting work on new projects, such as the sitter service in Brighton. This period gave him an insight into the need for simple written materials for workers who had little experience or qualifications. The result was the booklet *Working with Alzheimer's Disease*, which first appeared in 1988. It is now in its fifth edition and has also been published as a paperback. A companion booklet followed in 1990 – *Working alongside Carers* was based on the experience gained during two years as Training Officer for Care for the Carers in East Sussex.

David currently runs training courses for professionals and carers on dementia issues. He has set up his own publishing house called Ullswater Publications.

Acknowledgements

My thanks to the many carers of people with dementia whom I have met since 1984 and especially to Simon's mother who was prepared to let me write about her and her son. Thanks also go to the Alzheimer's Society. Without the help of the Society this book would have been very difficult to write. So thank you to Clive Evers who read the first version of the book and made many valuable suggestions for improvement; to Lesley MacKinnon, the Librarian; to Steve Milton in Information; and to others who helped me to find my way around the Library. Thank you also to Professor James Lindesay for commenting on the manuscript.

David Sutcliffe

Introduction

People over the age of 80 form the fastest growing group in the UK population today. The over-80s have the greatest risk of dementia, with about 20 per cent suffering from it in one form or another. Whilst some people with dementia manage without outside help, an increasing number need to be looked after by people who understand what is happening to the damaged brain and who are able to use an empathetic approach to them in their work.

This book is written for carers who are new to working with people with dementia. It is also intended to be useful to family carers who want to know more about dementia. It provides basic information about the condition, how it progresses, how it can be diagnosed and how the different types of dementia manifest themselves. Different approaches to care are discussed with a view to promoting a better understanding and quality of care through a person-centred approach. The book suggests that the key to successful working is through the understanding of what is happening to the person, looking beneath the 'problem' behaviour to the individual needs and feelings. It describes practical ways of helping people with dementia to have a sense of well-being. Examples are given throughout to illustrate the points being made. The key points are summarised at the end of each chapter.

The book concludes with a chapter which examines likely developments in the future. A glossary explains the terminology used and a list of useful addresses suggests sources for further information.

What is meant by dementia?

This chapter examines what happens to the brain when dementia sets in. It looks at the numbers of people with dementia in the UK, both young and old, and at their life expectancy. It then considers possible causes, highlighting the link to old age as well as family links, environmental factors and head injuries.

Loss of cells in the brain

Dementia is not a new form of illness; it has been with us for centuries. It is the name given to a range of conditions in which the brain goes through a long process of failure, beginning with a slight loss of memory and progressing to a total inability to cope with any aspect of life. There are a number of dementing illnesses, which are dealt with in Chapter 2. Some, like Alzheimer's disease, have become household names in the last decade, whilst others are very rare indeed.

The main feature is a loss of cells in the brain. We all lose cells as we get older but we have so many brain cells that the loss of a small percentage usually has no real effect on our life. However, in dementia the loss becomes catastrophic. In the earlier stages it is limited to a small section of the brain – for example in Alzheimer's disease it is the hippocampus (the memory bank) which is often the first part to be affected. As the disease advances, however, there is a more general shrinkage, with perhaps as much as one third of the total weight of the brain being lost. Losses continue to increase, so that one by one skills disappear and people with the illness become more and more confused. Eventually they may get to a terminal stage of the illness, at which point former skills, memory, and even personality, have more or less vanished.

Numbers of people with dementia

Dementia tends to be seen as inevitable, at least if you live long enough. The exceptions somehow seem to prove the rule. We agree that Bob, who lives on his own at the age of 95, is a living miracle, and that Polly is a marvel because she can recall events of long ago, and also those of yesterday. To our minds such skills are unusual and worth commenting on, when they are really only what we expect from everyone else. In reality, dementia only affects a minority of older people, leaving the vast majority with brains unaffected by such disease.

Prevalence (all ages)

Calculations of the numbers of people with dementia are based on prevalence rates as follows:

Age:		
	40–65	1 in 1,000
	65–70	1 in 50
	70–80	1 in 20
	80+	1 in 5

(Gray and Fenner 1993)

The pattern after the age of 90 is unclear. An extrapolation of the prevalence table would indicate that by the age of 100 everybody would suffer from dementia. We know, however, that this is not the case, as there are many people over 100 with no sign of dementia.

The total numbers in the UK are estimated at between 450,000 and 500,000, with a possible rise to over 650,000 in the first quarter of the 21st century (Bosanquet et al 1998). Even higher figures were quoted by the Alzheimer's Society in its evidence to the Royal Commission on Long-Term Care in 1998, namely 720,491 now, and 894,000 by the year 2021.

Prevalence by disease (all ages)

It is difficult to diagnose accurately the type of dementia that a person is suffering from. Lovestone (1998) has pointed to two factors which explain the complications of dementia diagnosis. Firstly there is a lack of, and need for, large-scale studies over a long period of time, starting in the community and finishing at post-mortem. The second issue is the fact that the diseases often do not exist in a pure form. For example, changes indicative of vascular disease are frequently found in patients with Alzheimer's disease and substantial vascular damage is found in the brains of older people with no dementing illness. As a result of his research Lovestone suggested two different sets of figures. Firstly, dementia as a single disorder, where his prevalence figures are:

Alzheimer's disease	55 per cent
Vascular dementia	20 per cent
Lewy-Body dementia	20 per cent
Others (including rare conditions, such as Creutzfeldt-Jakob Disease and Pick's Disease)	10 per cent

(Lovestone 1998)

Lovestone then gave figures for 'mixed disorders':

Alzheimer's disease only	40 per cent
Alzheimer's disease and vascular dementia	15 per cent
Alzheimer's disease and vascular damage	10 per cent
Vascular change	10 per cent
Other dementias and Alzheimer or vascular changes	10 per cent
Lewy-Body only	10 per cent
Lewy-Body and Alzheimer's disease	15 per cent

(Lovestone 1998)

Incidence of dementia

The incidence (new cases) of dementia also increases with age, from about 2 per 1,000 at age 65 to about 80 per 1,000 at age 90. About two-thirds of these new cases are of Alzheimer's disease (Launer et al 1999).

The younger person with dementia

The major risk factor which can lead to dementia is old age, with the prevalence rate doubling every five years after the age of 65.

At this older age dementia is sometimes known as late-onset (or, in the past, senile) dementia. This distinguishes it from early-onset (or, in the past, pre-senile) dementia, which describes people under 65. Those people who have a late-onset dementia are likely to have a slower version of the disease, and may well die of other conditions such as cancer or heart disease rather than because of an underlying dementia.

Alzheimer's disease can make an appearance as early as the age of 40. Although the percentage of people under retirement age who have dementia is insignificant, in all there are estimated to be 17,000 men and women in the UK with early-onset dementia. That seems a huge number, but from a GP's point of view it is rare enough for only a handful of cases to pass through the surgery doors in a lifetime of practising medicine, and it can therefore be very easy to mistake it for some other condition. For the families it can be a very isolating experience, as they may never come across anyone else with a similar condition and may have great problems with carrying on with normal life.

James was in his mid-40s when he started to have difficulties keeping up with the pace of work at his office. As a manager, he was able to delegate to his colleagues, and used his position of authority to fend off awkward questions. At home, he became increasingly unhelpful and withdrawn, which led to a number of serious arguments with his wife. Eventually, his poor performance at work came to the attention of his managers, who insisted that he visit his GP. The doctor diagnosed depression, but James did not respond to treatment and continued to deteriorate. A few months later, he stormed out of the house after yet another row with his wife, and did not return. He was found wandering the streets and was taken by the police to hospital. At this point his dementia was finally diagnosed. Two years on, he is now severely impaired, and is being looked after at home by his wife, who has had to give up her job and most of her social life in order to do this.

Pick's Disease is a dementia of the frontal lobe which can also attack as early as at 40 years of age. Creutzfeldt-Jakob Disease (CJD) can start in the 50s and 60s, whilst the new variant appears to mostly involve people under the age of 40, including teenagers. There are also a small but growing number of cases of AIDS-related dementia.

The percentage for each of the major dementias is given as follows in *Young-Onset Dementia* (Harvey 1998):

Alzheimer's disease	35 per cent
Fronto-temporal dementia	
(including Pick's Disease)	17 per cent
Vascular dementia	18 per cent
Alcohol-related dementia	13 per cent
Others	17 per cent

The 'others' category includes rarer forms of dementia, such as AIDS-related dementia, Huntington's Chorea and multiple sclerosis.

Life expectancy of people with dementia

The life expectancy of someone with dementia is difficult to determine. Death rates in studies give huge variations (as much as 45 per cent difference). For some younger people, dementia may run its course in as little as five years. With older people, it may be eight or ten years or even more. The length of time that people live with dementia varies widely and also depends on the sort of dementia involved. In practice many older people die of other conditions, such as cancer, before the dementing illness can get to the final stage. Where it does become a terminal illness, death is likely to be caused by some condition like bronchio pneumonia which is brought on by the fact that patients are immobile and unable to swallow or to look after themselves properly. In general, good standards of care lead to longer life expectancy.

Possible causes

Dementia is linked to old age

Dementia is talked about a lot more today – that is true at least of Alzheimer's disease and CJD. The question is often posed as to whether we are bringing illness upon ourselves by the way we live. The truth is that dementia is in general linked to age. Since people are living longer, it is not surprising that dementia is on the increase. Many people who are over 80 today would have had little chance of reaching their 60th birthday in the past – the rise of dementia goes hand in hand with rising living standards in the developed world.

Vascular dementia has a known cause – small strokes which can be controlled through the use of aspirin. Apart from alcohol-related dementias, however, other conditions like Alzheimer's disease and Pick's Disease have no known cause. There is a range of possibilities, including faulty genes or an environmental trigger.

The family link

Each of us has 46 chromosomes which are the blueprint for each of the cells in our body. They are paired, and numbered from 1 to 22, with the last pair being the sex chromosomes. Some genes, however, may be faulty and are the cause of certain conditions which can lead to inherited illnesses. They can also give us a higher than average (or lower than average) risk of contracting an illness.

There is a tiny number of families in the world which have a defective gene on either chromosome 14 or 21 which results in a trail of Alzheimer's disease through the generations. People who fall ill in these families tend to be younger (between 35 and 60) than the so-called 'sporadic' cases.

More common are genes which can alter the risk of developing the illness. We all have a copy of one of three types of a protein called Apolipoprotein E; if we have two copies of the E4 version, we have an increased risk of getting Alzheimer's disease. As old age is a major risk factor as well, very old people who have the ApoE4 gene are very likely to develop the illness, especially if they have inherited the ApoE4 gene from both their parents. On the other hand, the E2 version gives protection from Alzheimer's disease.

In Down's Syndrome there is an extra copy of chromosome 21, which also carries one of the genes which, if faulty, leads to Alzheimer's disease in a small number of families. As a result most people with Down's Syndrome develop Alzheimer's disease if they live long enough. American research in 1989 suggested that 6 per cent of people with Down's Syndrome in their 30s have Alzheimer's disease, with the figure rising to 75 per cent for those over the age of 55 (Holland 1993). In most cases the cause of damage is the deposition of the protein β-amyloid (beta-amyloid – see page 12).

Environmental factors

Aluminium was once thought to be an important cause of dementia, and there was a rapid clear-out of aluminium pans in some households. Although there is evidence of aluminium deposits in the brains of people who have died of Alzheimer's disease, that is no different from other 'healthy' brains. It is conceivable that some water supplies may contain too much aluminium, but there do not appear to be clusters of dementia in areas of the country where there is a lot of aluminium in the water supply. Today most scientists believe that the aluminium deposits are a by-product of dementia, not a cause of it.

Mercury is another chemical which has been targeted, especially in connection with amalgam fillings in dentistry. Other chemicals may poison both brain and body – organo-phosphates, for example, which are claimed to be the cause of Gulf War Syndrome and some unexplained illnesses among farm workers. Dementia, of course, pre-dates both mercury fillings and organo-phosphates.

Head injury

Another possible cause is related to a previous head injury. As with Down's Syndrome, the protein β-amyloid is implicated as the cause of the damage. There is evidence that this protein is laid down very quickly after a serious head injury, such as one incurred as the result of a fall down the stairs, a car crash, or a bad skiing injury for example. It could also be the explanation for dementia in ex-boxers who have put themselves in the position of having brain injuries similar to those who have had accidents. Other sports may have similar effects. It has for example been suggested that footballers may be putting themselves at risk when they head footballs coming at them at high speed.

β-amyloid is gradually deposited in the brain as people get older. So its presence does not by itself indicate that a person will develop dementia.

Key points

■ In dementia the brain fails progressively.

■ There is a range of illnesses under the heading of dementia.

■ People over the age of 70 are at greater risk.

■ One in five people over the age of 80 suffer from dementia.

■ In the UK there are 17,000 younger people with dementia (that is, under the age of 65).

■ Dementia is becoming more common because people are living longer.

■ The causes of dementia are not yet fully understood (except in vascular dementia).

■ The risk to some people is a genetic one. People with Down's Syndrome are very likely to develop Alzheimer's disease.

■ Previous head injury may increase the risk of developing dementia.

CHAPTER 2

Types of dementia

Alzheimer's disease

The main form of dementia is named after Alois Alzheimer. This section describes the features of the brain which he discovered and draws on more recent research. It explains the problem that some of the features found in the brains of those with Alzheimer's disease are also found in the brains of people who have not had dementia. It looks at possible causes, risk factors and also at some factors which are believed to offer protection. Clinical signs of illness are examined and the section concludes by examining the progression of the disease in people with dementia and the implications of the cost of the new drugs.

Alzheimer's original research

Alzheimer's disease has become a well-known disease. It used to be seen as an illness which was very rare, a condition of 'younger' people, which a doctor might see once or twice in a career. Such 'younger' people showed signs of ageing whilst still in middle life, a senility which was only unusual because the person with the illness was only 45 or 50. It used to be known as *pre-senile dementia*, to distinguish it from *senile dementia*. Today we realise that Alzheimer's is a common disease of older people, and also one which attacks a small but significant group of younger men and women.

It was in 1906 that Alois Alzheimer did his original research. He was one of several researchers all working on the problem of why some people showed signs of premature ageing. He studied in particular the brain of a woman who had died aged 51 after years of illness. He noted three things:

1 What he described as neuro-fibrillary tangles
2 Loss of brain cells in the cortex
3 Senile plaques made of a substance called *amyloid*

To Alzheimer these were indications of an ageing process which had started in middle life, giving rise to the idea that it could be described as a pre-senile condition. His colleague Emil Kraepelin, however, saw the illness as something unique which was not linked to the age of the person. The Alzheimer view would suggest that everyone develops dementia if they live long enough. We have seen, however, that although the number of people with dementia increases after the age of 80 in particular (see page 2), there are many very old people with no sign of dementia even at the end of their lives. Over the years the 'Kraepelin' view of the disease has been generally more accepted than that of Alzheimer himself. Yet nobody was able to say what the cause of the disease was. There were, however, a number of theories which were put forward at various times.

Theories about causes

A genetic problem

The big fear for many people in middle age is that they are going to suffer from Alzheimer's just as a parent may have done. In fact for some people there are family members in various generations who have had a form of dementia. Some families have a genetic fault which leads to early-onset Alzheimer's, but these are small in number (see page 6). In most other cases any genetic cause merely increases risk. In other words, the chances of getting Alzheimer's disease increase, but still the main risk factor is old age.

Old age

The biggest risk factor is age (a one in five chance at age 80+).

More women than men

There are more women than men with Alzheimer's disease, but there are suggestions from some studies that this is only true in late-onset cases.

Injuries to the head

Head injuries result in the deposition of amyloid during the immediate period after the accident. Some, but not all, studies have indicated a positive link with dementia afterwards (see page 7).

Education

Some studies have indicated that a higher standard of education is a protection against Alzheimer's disease. However, poor education may be masking other areas of poverty which assist the development of Alzheimer's disease (Burns et al 1995).

Smoking

Some studies have indicated that there is a protective factor in nicotine, and that therefore smoking could be seen as a protective factor against dementia. However, smoking is a risk factor for vascular diseases, including multi-infarct dementia.

The threshold theory

'The straw that breaks the camel's back' may prove to be the final cause of Alzheimer's disease. Losses in the brain may not affect daily living until there have been so many of them that the disease is triggered. This is similar to the situation with Parkinson's Disease, where as many as 85 per cent of cells have to be lost before there are clinical signs of the illness. The same certainly applies to multi-infarct dementia, where there has to be a series of small strokes before the onset of dementia.

Changes in the brain

Senile plaques

The plaques described by Alzheimer are lesions (damage to brain tissue) with a centre made of the poisonous protein amyloid. These are found in the hippocampus at the base of the brain and in the neocortex (the main outer mass of the brain). There is a correlation between the amount of plaque and the severity of the dementia condition. However, senile plaques may be present in the brains of people with no history of dementia.

Amyloid protein is also called β-amyloid (beta-amyloid) and β-A4 peptide. It comes from a larger protein called amyloid precursor protein (APP). Burns et al (1995) indicate that it is an early feature of Alzheimer's disease. The protein is toxic to neurones. Current research into drug treatments is targeting the APP in the expectation that an alteration in its metabolism could slow down the deposition of β-amyloid.

Neuro-fibrillary tangles

These are twisted molecules made of protein which are found within the nerve cells and are implicated in the losses in the brains of people with Alzheimer's disease. They cause a degeneration of the neurones, and are a cause of the dying of cells in the brain and an accompanying loss of brain function. However, they also occur in the brains of other older people who do not have signs of dementia.

Tau protein is connected with the neuro-fibrillary tangles. It is a late feature of the disease and is, like β-amyloid, an abnormal protein. We all have the normal form, which is soluble. In Alzheimer's disease tau becomes insoluble and increases in amount, by up to 19 times, causing neurones to die. The amount of tau correlates closely with the clinical signs of Alzheimer's disease in the patient.

Impaired neurotransmission

Nerve cells in the brain communicate by means of chemical messengers called neurotransmitters. In Alzheimer's disease, as the cells die, there is a steady reduction in the levels of some of these neurotransmitters. In particular, there is loss of cells that communicate using the chemical acetylcholine. As parts of the chemical system involving acetylcholine are unaffected by the disease, drug treatments have been developed to increase the amount of the chemical and enable the development of the disease to be delayed. This is the basis of treatment available as a result of the first round of drugs to be licensed in the UK (Aricept and Exelon – see pages 16–17).

In addition, there are low levels of other neurotransmitters, especially noradrenalin, serotonin and dopamine (the latter being identified as deficient in Parkinson's Disease).

Clinical signs

The slow, insidious nature of the illness at the outset makes it very difficult for anyone to be sure when Alzheimer's disease has begun its course. People with dementia can be expert in covering up their problems even from their nearest and dearest, so that it can be a great shock to family and friends when the truth comes to light and they realise how bad the dementia has become. Eventually there will be indications that all is not well. The most likely sign will be a failure of memory, an inability to remember names, or perhaps an incident where the person gets lost unexpectedly. Gaps in both knowledge and skills will become apparent.

Loss of memory

Memory of recent events may be damaged, with earlier memories retained. Eventually events in the more distant past are wiped out as well.

Loss of language skills

There is a huge range of language problems, including:

- apparent nonsense speech;
- repeating the last word or sound said by someone else; and
- an inability to find a noun or name.

Forgetting a second language may cause problems for people living in an adopted country. However, there is evidence of the development of a poetic language, which can be hard for carers to make sense of. In the final stages of the illness there may be no language left, or just words like 'yes' or 'no'. (See pages 48–51 for further information.)

Spatial skills

Spatial skills (a sense of space) include being able to dress correctly or to set the table. Without help, people with Alzheimer's disease are unlikely to be able to cope with a range of activities of daily life. They may find it hard to locate the chair to sit down on, miss it and find themselves on the floor alongside the chair. One useful diagnostic test involves asking people to copy a simple diagram, for example a small house. For people with Alzheimer's disease (and other dementias) it may prove to be very difficult to do.

Inability to recognise things

This covers a range of skill losses, including:

● inability to read, write or calculate;
● inability to identify an everyday object, such as a watch or a cup, without looking at it; and
● inability to identify faces correctly.

Personality changes

There may be changes in habit. For example, a person who always dressed well may become extremely untidy or vice versa. There may be a loss of tact and a removal of the inhibitions which were learned as a child. This change may lead to difficult behaviour in public, such as goods being taken from the local shop, or sexual disinhibition (removal of clothing, masturbation in public etc). Burns et al (1995) talk of three main features:

● a reduction of interests;
● adoption of rigid stereotyped routines; and
● sudden explosion of emotion when taxed beyond their restricted ability (catastrophic reaction).

Medical explanations do not take into consideration the individuality of the person who has Alzheimer's disease. Kitwood's alternative concept is that dementing illnesses should be seen, primarily, as forms of disability

(Kitwood 1995). With this model, how a person is affected depends crucially on the quality of care. Instead of seeing Alzheimer's as an illness to be managed, it suggests that the emphasis should be on understanding the person in the midst of their changing world. It questions the way in which 'normal' people set the agenda; that is, whether the needs of disabled (dementing) people are properly taken into consideration in the house or the care home or the workplace. Unusual behaviour may not be the result of a changed personality so much as an attempt to cope with frightening situations.

> **Ethel** is blind and suffers from severe dementia; she now lives in a nursing home. Her GP was called because she was hitting out at the staff during meals and at bathtimes. They asked if she could be given some medication to 'calm her down'. The GP in turn referred her to the local old age psychiatrist, who came to assess her. On questioning the staff, it became apparent that they were delivering Ethel's care without any warning or explanation. Because she could not see or understand what was happening, she thought she was being assaulted and reacted accordingly.

Concentrating on the losses, on what a person is unable to do leads to a negative view of the person. Improvement comes by looking at what people with dementia can do. It is necessary to have a view of a unique individual who will need help to overcome the difficulties that dementia puts in the way. Chapter 4 (see pages 80–92) looks at ways in which care staff can highlight those areas which are still a person's strength, and make use of them.

Psychotic symptoms

Psychotic symptoms in dementia can include hallucinations, delusions and paranoia. The medical explanation is that these mood changes are a feature of the disease. However, since people with Alzheimer's disease have difficulties in making sense of their world, an inability to perceive the world correctly may result in a false interpretation which others consider evidence for paranoia. The claim that the boys are playing on the roof may be something to do with the central heating making noises. The hallucinations may go away when the television is turned off and care staff relate to the individual's own needs for attention and emotional support.

Progression of the disease

People with Alzheimer's disease usually show a steady decline in the course of their illness. This is in contrast to the more step-like pattern of vascular (multi-infarct) dementia (see page 20) and the erratic pattern of Lewy-Body dementia (see page 23).

A 'stage' view of dementia predominated until recently, with certain deficits being linked to early, middle and late stages. Individuals do not, however, always conform to the average or usual pattern of decline. Bell and McGregor (1995) have outlined seven dangers of adopting a stage theory of dementia:

● It can be a self-fulfilling prophecy.
● It shifts the emphasis away from the individual with specific problems.
● It limits people's opportunities to realise their true potential.
● It dehumanises the person.
● It offers a hopeless future of inevitable decline.
● It allows no scope for innovation or progress.
● It lowers the status of both the person and the care staff.

At the final (terminal) point, the person will have lost a lot of weight and may be in bed, perhaps in the foetal position. There may be no response, although that does not mean that the person cannot hear. Death may have several possible causes, including an inability to swallow (death follows as the person gets weaker) or a chest infection (people with Alzheimer's disease are less able to fight off the infection). Death certificates may sometimes give Alzheimer's disease as one of the causes of death. It is, however, only an underlying cause, and may not be recognised by the doctor as being important enough to include on the certificate.

Many people with Alzheimer's disease die from other conditions, such as heart disease and cancer. For such people there is concern that they may not receive enough pain control in the terminal stage, as they may be unable to identify pain correctly or to tell anyone how they are feeling.

Anti-Alzheimer drugs

The new drugs (*Aricept* and *Exelon*) allow a modification of the decline seen in Alzheimer's in many, but not all, patients, when given in the early stages of the illness. Neither drug is a cure for Alzheimer's disease. They can delay the development of the disease in some people who are at an early stage. For example in studies of treatment using Exelon, the best results showed a slight improvement up to week 40, followed by gradual decline.

The cost of anti-Alzheimer drugs

Most drugs are free on the NHS. When Aricept arrived in 1997, it took most health authorities by surprise and challenged their budgets. To begin with only eight authorities authorised the use of Aricept, but, by 1998, with the arrival of Exelon, many other authorities developed their own protocols for prescribing.

Since specialists in most health authorities were unable to prescribe at first, some carers used their own money to provide for the person they were looking after. However, other Alzheimer drugs will arrive on the market, and the Government will need to deal with the extra cost to the NHS which this implies so as to ensure that people with Alzheimer's disease are not denied treatment on the grounds of cost. Clearly there have to be limits, but decisions about resources should not be permitted to result in a two-tier Alzheimer care programme in which only those with money could take advantage of the available drugs. The National Institute for Clinical Excellence (NICE) will be looking at the issue of anti-Alzheimer drugs in 2001.

Key points

■ Alois Alzheimer conducted his research in 1906 on middle-aged people who showed signs of premature ageing.

■ Risk factors for developing Alzheimer's include: old age; a genetic link; or a head injury.

■ The threshold theory asserts that a build-up of many 'causes' eventually results in triggering dementia.

- The signs within the brain include: senile plaques; neuro-fibrillary tangles; and the loss of some chemicals.

- Clinical signs include: memory loss; loss of language skills; problems with sense of space; and an inability to recognise things and people.

- The pattern of decline varies according to the individual.

- The costs of the new drugs are high and some patients are paying for their prescriptions.

Other dementias

Dementia can be caused by a series of mini-strokes, which may not have been obvious to others. This type of dementia is called 'vascular' or 'multi-infarct' (MID). The damage may be confined to one area of the brain and so the losses may be very limited at the beginning. This section deals with its step-like progress and the fact that it can be prevented with the use of aspirin. Other less common dementias examined include Pick's Disease, Lewy-Body Disease, alcohol-related dementia (Korsakoff's Syndrome) and the prion diseases, the best known of which is CJD.

Multi-infarct dementia (MID)

Vascular disease can lead to dementia, either suddenly following a stroke or over time through a series of small strokes in the brain. The latter is called multi-infarct dementia or MID and generally occurs in later life. The strokes cause damage to the brain, but, unlike major strokes, may not be obvious at the time. People may appear to have just dropped off to sleep for a short while, and to have woken up again in a normal manner, or they may experience dizziness. However, there may be situations where the effects of a mini-stroke are evident, as in the following three cases:

Margaret's handwriting was always beautiful. It reflected the style of the school that she had attended long ago. One evening she was writing her diary as usual, when she had a tiny stroke. Nobody noticed and she herself just thought that she had fallen asleep for a short while, but her special handwriting style had changed. Although it was still legible, there was a definite change that could be seen in the middle of the entry for that day. There was no great emergency, no doctor needed to be called, but it was another step on the way to the dementia that Margaret was to develop in the next few months.

Gordon went to the theatre with his daughter one afternoon. Suddenly he keeled over in his seat and went unconscious for a moment. In a few minutes he was being whisked away through the traffic to the casualty department of the nearest hospital. By the time they had got there, Gordon had recovered and was wondering out loud what the fuss was all about. To make sure there was nothing seriously wrong, they kept him in hospital for a couple of days to have some tests.

John drove his car into the wall as he was manoeuvring in front of the house. The front of the car was quite badly damaged. The wall crashed into the neighbour's flower bed and damaged his prize roses. John could not understand what had happened. He was persuaded (with considerable difficulty) that he should stop driving altogether, and his wife sold the car to make sure that he wasn't tempted to set off in it again. Dementia began to take hold of John about a year later.

Symptoms

Many of the symptoms of MID are similar to those of Alzheimer's disease. There may be the same problems of wandering and the same loss of skills. Some people may be able to give the appearance that all is completely well, as very little of the brain has been affected. However, the loss of certain skills may result in the person not being able to look after themself properly any longer. If, for example, you have forgotten the sequences used in cooking, then it is no longer easy to live an independent life. If you have no idea about using the toilet, it may mean the end of any social life whatsoever. Eventually such problems may make it necessary for the person to be admitted to full-time care. Some of the earlier signs of MID are urinary incontinence and also difficulties with walking, both of which may lead to an early loss of independence.

Progression of the disease

The disease follows a step-like pattern of decline; ie decline follows a small stroke (although not necessarily every small stroke). These steps do not occur at regular intervals, so there is no way of determining the course of the disease. Some people survive with low levels of dementia for many years, and do not suffer further brain losses.

Prevention

Of all the dementias MID is the only one which can at present be prevented. As with other stroke conditions, it is linked to high blood pressure, and can therefore be affected by such factors as diet, exercise and smoking. Removing animal fat from the diet, stopping smoking and taking regular exercise can thus help to reduce the chance of developing this type of dementia. Aspirin is also used as a preventative (at the GP's suggestion).

Stroke

Strokes occur when the brain suffers an obstruction or a burst blood vessel. Most people who survive a stroke do not usually suffer from dementia; instead they are likely to have speech and movement losses. However, one person in five is left with some mental damage or confusion. In these cases it is not known whether there was the beginning of an Alzheimer condition which was suddenly accelerated by the stroke, or whether it was just the effects of a stroke on its own.

Fronto-temporal dementia

Whilst Alzheimer's disease attacks the hippocampus and then brings about a gradual shrinkage of the brain, fronto-temporal dementia targets the frontal lobes. This means that the area of our brain that deals with mood and behaviour begins to suffer from a loss of cells. The result is like a ship that has lost its steering. The person with fronto-temporal dementia is aware of the deficit, and is likely to be even more frustrated than the person with Alzheimer's. One reason for this is the early onset of the disease – usually before the age of 60. People who are still working may realise that they are not performing at the level that they should and are likely to devise strategies for coping. Some of these strategies will be designed to keep others from finding out the truth. They may become more secretive and they may also delegate tasks which they know that they cannot do any longer.

Symptoms

The major form of fronto-temporal dementia is Pick's Disease. Anger and aggression are often the hallmarks of the illness, and can alienate friends, neighbours and fellow workers. There will also be bouts of apathy and behaviour patterns which bring dismay and confusion to others. Sometimes there will be a loss of tact in conversation or behaviour which is eccentric to the point of giving offence.

The symptoms are such that they are unlikely to be recognised as illness to start with. They may be seen just as unreasonable behaviour and trigger off a crisis such as a marriage breakdown, leaving the person with the illness even more isolated and vulnerable than would have been the case anyway. Alternatively it may be viewed as a mental health or alcohol-related problem.

Simon is in his late 40s. His dementia symptoms were first noticed about seven years ago and he was admitted to hospital over Christmas as it was thought that he was suffering from a brain tumour. His behaviour had become quite volatile, and he was unable to cope with his work as a freelance writer. Heavy drinking led the hospital to diagnose Korsakoff's Syndrome, which at least gave a name to the illness, but did nothing for Simon's future. At this point his wife rejected him altogether, and he became the responsibility of his mother who lived about 50 miles away. Simon moved into a bedsit, but was not able to look after himself properly. Finance was a problem with an insurance company refusing to pay out on an income protection policy. As Korsakoff's is a condition caused by alcohol, the insurance company claimed that the illness was self-inflicted and outside the terms of the policy. The hasty diagnosis was now a label which would take four years to remove. Living alone became gradually more and more risky, and Simon's mother took the decision to look after him herself. Simon's worsening condition indicated that Korsakoff's was an incorrect diagnosis. It seemed to be an unknown mental illness, which could be treated socially. A psychiatric day centre did not prove helpful. His mother's insistence on a further referral locally led to the diagnosis of *pre-senile dementia*. Brain scans a year apart brought the news that the disease was a frontal lobe dementia, probably Pick's Disease.

Simon needed to be watched all the time, as he was likely to take things belonging to other patients. There are few specialist homes with staff trained to look after such a young person and respite care in the local hospital was inappropriate. A move to assess him elsewhere lasted less than a day, before he was returned to the hospital by the assessment unit which could not cope with Simon's behaviour. In hospital he began to be incontinent and was on the receiving end of violent behaviour by other patients in the ward.

Simon's continued stay in the local hospital was largely caused by the inability of the health authorities to agree on who should pay for him. Eventually, after advice from the Community Health Council and a carers support group, the money was made available for him to be looked after in a specialist hospital and the transfer was carried out sensitively. His mother was able to make the 30-mile journey regularly to visit him and the insurance company was persuaded to listen to the proper diagnosis and pay the money that it owed under the income protection policy.

As can be seen from Simon's story, diagnosis is very difficult. Pick's Disease and other fronto-temporal dementias are rare, and it is therefore easy to attribute symptoms to Alzheimer's disease or to a mental health problem instead.

Diffuse Lewy-Body Disease

Lewy-Body Disease may account for as much as 20 per cent of the total number of cases of dementia. It is, however, relatively unknown even among health workers. In many respects it is similar to Alzheimer's, but there are significant differences in its symptoms, and at post-mortem there are signs of unusual deposits in the brain. These deposits contain damaged nerve cells; they are known as 'Lewy bodies', and are named after the doctor who discovered them.

Symptoms

The special symptoms are the Parkinsonian traits, including the shakiness of hands, and stiffness of legs, which can lead to falls. People with Lewy-Body Disease also have difficulties in dealing with distances. They may find it difficult to judge the width of a doorway or they may not know exactly where a seat is located and appear to choose to sit on the floor alongside the chair. Some mistakes may cause no more than embarrassment, but there may be falls which cause real damage.

A further feature of Lewy-Body Disease is hallucinations. People with the disease may see people who are not present, or perhaps believe that there are people coming out of the television set. These can be symptoms of other forms of mental illness and also of Alzheimer's disease. Other signs of the illness include a low level of attention, confusion and a lack of verbal fluency.

Progression

Unlike Alzheimer's disease where decline is gradual, and vascular dementia where it is step-like, Lewy-Body Disease has an erratic pattern, with improvements as well as some days of steep decline. Overall the decline is at about the same rate as with Alzheimer's disease.

There is a link with Parkinson's Disease, as these same Lewy bodies are found in another area of the brain of people who have Parkinson's but have no sign of any dementia. It is important that they are not given certain tranquillising drugs which have serious side effects which do not occur in people with Alzheimer's disease. For this reason it is very important for the person with Lewy-Body Disease to be properly diagnosed.

Diagnosis

Diagnosis can be made more difficult by the fact that many people with the disease also have Alzheimer's disease. Gauthier has suggested that Lewy-Body and Alzheimer lesions interact to produce dementia (Gauthier 1996). An exact diagnosis is not possible until after death, but the presence of Parkinson-type features should at least alert doctors to the need to avoid tranquillising drugs. As with most other dementias, neither cause nor cure are known.

Huntington's Disease

Huntington's Disease is a form of dementia which is entirely hereditary. It attacks between the ages of 35 and 55 and is sometimes known as Huntington's Chorea, a term which describes the involuntary movements or contortions that the patient makes. Barely noticeable at the outset, there is a gradual slowing down of movements, a lack of rhythm, slow eye movements and poor balance. As the disease progresses, balance and walking become more and more difficult until the person is incapable of moving by themselves. Eye movements slow down and eventually stop altogether. Most people with Huntington's Disease develop dementia, but this is not always the case.

Korsakoff's Syndrome

Korsakoff's Syndrome is a rare dementia which is linked to alcoholism. Generally in dementia the disease gets worse, either gradually, or in a step-like fashion. In Korsakoff's Syndrome abstinence from alcohol stops the progress of the disease, but a large part of the memory bank is lost. Sacks tells the story of a man described as '*The Lost Mariner*'. This man had lost about 30 years of his memory and was firmly fixed at the end of the Second World War. Jimmie thought that he would be 20 next birthday and was shocked at what he saw when he was asked to look in a mirror. He was baffled by the experience, but it was a passing difficulty as he immediately forgot what had troubled him. He fitted into the description given by Korsakoff in 1887:

> 'Memory of recent events is disturbed almost exclusively; recent impressions apparently disappear soonest, whereas impressions of long ago are recalled properly, so that the patient's ingenuity, his sharpness of wit, and his resourcefulness remain largely unaffected.'
> (Sacks 1985)

This condition may be as distressing as any dementia, but, as long as alcohol is avoided, there is no further damage. A tiny area of the brain has been destroyed, leaving the rest intact. Jimmie was able to play games and puzzles, as long as they were played quickly enough for his limited memory span.

Prion diseases

Prions are infectious proteins which affect a tiny number of people around the world, most of whom are in the 45–75 age group. Only a small number of these illnesses are inherited. Prion diseases have the power to mutate; ie they can alter in nature as they pass from one person or group to another, and also from one species to another. The main prion disease in humans is Creutzfeldt-Jakob Disease (CJD).

CJD

There are usually less than 50 cases of CJD a year in the UK. It is thus a very rare disease that most of us will never encounter. However, it has become a household name as a result of its 'new variant' form which is linked to 'mad cow disease' and the beef crisis which followed in the 1990s.

Symptoms of the illness include headaches and weight loss, mental deterioration, depression and uncoordinated movements. It is a 'spongiform' dementia, which means that the brain takes on a sponge-like texture – in most dementias there is a loss of brain cells and a resultant loss of weight of the brain. The incubation period in humans can be long but compared to Alzheimer's disease, the course of the actual illness is rapid (ie from six months to three years from diagnosis).

Whilst most cases of CJD have an unknown cause, there have been examples of infection through medical treatment. There were cases of people receiving infected tissue as a result of cornea grafts and also young people were in some cases given hormone growth treatment which was similarly infected. Procedures have now been altered so that there is no longer any danger of this recurring.

CJD (new variant)

The new variant (version) of CJD is probably caused through eating infected beef products, or perhaps through contact with infected animals. The source of the infection is thought to be cows with BSE (Bovine Spongiform Encalopathy), popularly known as 'mad cow disease'. The number of deaths in Britain is 80 at present (Guardian, 28 October 2000) but the long incubation period means that it may be several decades before we can know the final total. Most victims have been young, with ages ranging from 13 to 40. However, a 74-year-old man died of the disease in October 2000, and this case, together with the overall rise in the number of cases, has prompted government experts to start to reassess the scale of the epidemic. Diagnosis is difficult, both because of the rarity of the illness, and also because the early symptoms are similar to signs of depression.

Key points

■ Strokes can lead to dementia, especially a series of mini-strokes which can remove certain skills. This is known as multi-infarct dementia (MID).

■ Pick's Disease is the major dementia affecting the frontal lobes of the brain. It tends to affect younger people.

■ Lewy-Body Disease has features akin to those of Parkinson's Disease, especially tremor and stiffness, and is similar to Alzheimer's disease.

■ Huntington's Disease is genetically transmitted, attacks people in middle life, and is distinguished by the way in which the limbs become contorted.

■ Korsakoff's Syndrome is a rare dementia linked to alcohol abuse.

■ Prion diseases are very rare infectious diseases, the best known of which is CJD. The new variant of CJD is a mutation which is thought to be linked to BSE ('mad cow disease').

'Curable' or containable conditions

Some symptoms give the impression that a person is suffering from some form of dementia when they have a condition that can be cured. This section looks at the effects of drugs, poor diet and the misuse of alcohol, as well as those of some illnesses and brain injuries. Temporary confusion (sometimes called 'delirium') can be mistaken for the early stages of dementia, as can the symptoms of depression. When the basic cause of these conditions is dealt with, the dementia goes. There are a range of other causes which may require the skills of an expert, such as an old age psychiatrist, if a proper diagnosis is to be made.

• •

Confusion

There used to be homes for 'the confused elderly', catering for people suffering from dementia. The label gave rise to the idea that confusion was in itself an illness. Of course it can describe the behaviour of people who have a dementing illness, but it is a very good description of everybody at some time or another. If we are put in a position of stress or given too many things to do at the same time, it is quite possible that we will fail to cope with daily activities. We may for example find ourselves on the train going in the wrong direction or turn up at the meeting a week early, or our frustrations may lead us to be angry over trifling annoyances. Confusion is a part of the healthy brain's activity as well as a sign that someone is suffering from dementia.

Alternatively confusion may be the result of a lack of concentration. The message never really reaches the brain, and as a result it can be easy to make a mistake, such as leaving a shop without paying for something at the checkout.

Confusion is also a major factor in the lives of people who have a form of dementia. They may find it difficult to remember where they are living; they may mistake a grandchild for their own child; they may imagine that they are going to work when in practice they are heading for the day centre. Confusion may be an accurate description of someone's behaviour and understanding, but it should never be used as a diagnosis.

Too many drugs

Doctors are careful about offering treatments which may cause problems of their own, but it is still possible for them to give too many different drugs to their patients. Different doctors in different places may prescribe without proper communication; the result can be a combination of medicines which leads to a state of confusion which can be easily mistaken for dementia. An older person may forget that they have taken a drug, so they take a second dose. Confusion begins to take more of a hold and they take yet another dose; they may become unable to function properly and start giving signs that they are failing in mind as well as in body.

Unmonitored drug combinations may result in a range of side effects and adverse interactions which lead to a decline in awareness and in brain function. It may not be the doctor's fault – it could merely be that a drug bought over the counter for a cold might not interact well with another prescription drug which is regularly used for a physical condition. Drugs and alcohol do not make a good mixture, and some older people have nobody around to keep an eye on them and prevent them from having their usual glass of beer when the medicine bottle states that alcohol should not be taken with the drug. Those drugs that target the central nervous system, such as tranquillisers, are relevant in this respect, but there is also a huge range of prescribed drugs which cause drowsiness in the general public, such as some antibiotics and antihistamines for example.

With medical advice and supervision, the person can be weaned off a drug in order to see if there is an improvement in alertness; it is vital, however, that drugs are not just removed from patients without medical advice and also without good monitoring of their condition. There are also ways of helping people to remember to take only one dose at a time; one example is a container designed to dispense pills on a regular basis.

Illnesses and injury

Joan was found by her next-door neighbour slumped in the armchair of her living room. She had not been seen all weekend and the neighbour had begun to get worried when there were no signs of life on Monday morning. The kitchen was in a terrible mess with bits of food all over the place. Joan's clothes were soaked in urine; she had tried to get to the toilet, but had not made it in time, so there were faeces up the stairs. The neighbour was stunned, as Joan was always so clean and tidy. The thought of dementia ran through her mind, but fortunately the doctor had no difficulty in diagnosing a simple case of bronchitis.

Bronchitis can cause confusion in older people, as can both urinary tract infections and constipation. Whilst younger people recover without much sign of confusion, older people may be struck down by temporary incontinence, they may be unable to speak coherently or they may have some loss of memory. However, with good care and attention, a dose of antibiotics and plenty of fluids, the symptoms will vanish within a few days, and the 'dementia' will pass away.

An abnormal thyroid condition may give the impression of a dementia. Usually this is caused by an under-active thyroid gland and the symptoms go away when the underlying condition has been controlled.

Brain damage

Brain tumours can produce symptoms that make both families and medical staff think that dementia has started. For some people a brain tumour can cause aggression and can seem to change the whole personality. Brain lesions (damage to brain tissue) can occur after a head injury and result in blood collecting in the space between two of the coverings of the brain. As with tumours, this causes pressure to build up in the brain and creates symptoms which are similar to dementia. This can happen at any age, but is relatively easy to diagnose if the condition is linked to a recent fall. More difficult is the chronic version which involves a slow build-up of blood as a result of a minor knock on the head or even a sudden jerk which goes unnoticed by other people. People who have this chronic condition are usually over 60, and may well present with symptoms which are easily mistaken for Alzheimer's disease.

Fortunately brain scans (for example Magnetic Resonance Imaging) have made it easier to see the difference between the various forms of lesions and diseases such as Alzheimer's. Surgery can offer a return to normality in many cases, and in others the swelling can be reduced by means of drugs.

Poor diet

We may think that malnutrition in developed countries is a thing of the past, but some people who live on their own are at risk of having an inadequate diet. They may get out of the habit of cooking properly when there is nobody else there to cook for. They may have a reduced appetite and just not enjoy their food any more. Limited finances may lead them to cut costs by skipping meals altogether. They may even be more concerned to see that the cat gets enough to eat and neglect their own needs. A balanced diet is a necessity for all of us, if we are to remain healthy, but there are two particular elements in our diet which are needed if we are to avoid the signs of dementia.

First of all we need vitamin B12. This is in fortified cereals and also in liver. Secondly we need zinc, which is a mineral found in many common foods. A poor diet is likely to be deficient in one or other of these two important elements and a cause of the confusional states which mimic dementia. A folic acid deficiency does not usually occur on its own, but is associated with a lack of vitamin B12. However, there have been cases of dementia without a lack of vitamin B12, which have been responsive to folate therapy. Someone who is deficient in vitamin B12 normally needs a series of injections to redress the balance.

Alcohol

In people who are dependent on alcohol, sudden withdrawal can produce a range of symptoms which mimic those of dementia. Loss of mental function, forgetfulness, hallucinations, and even a condition known as delirium tremens (the DTs), can all look remarkably similar to the problems of people with Alzheimer's disease, but they are likely to clear up in most cases within a few days. However, hardened older drinkers may eventually begin to have a more chronic form of dementia, known as alcohol-related dementia. Stopping drinking may arrest the decline, but there may be damage to the frontal lobes (the management area) of the brain (Harvey 1998). As a result it becomes more difficult for the person to steer clear of alcohol, and the condition then gets worse, with a pattern of slow decline. (See also page 24 on Korsakoff's Syndrome.)

Depression

It can be difficult to determine whether a person is suffering from depression or the early stages of dementia. Superficially the symptoms can appear to be the same. There may be a loss of cognitive function (ie damage to the person's ability to learn, reason and solve problems), combined with reduced awareness of people and places. The symptoms may disappear as a result of treatment. However, it is not surprising when people in the early stages of dementia are aware enough of their problems and mental decline to feel depressed about their situation.

Key points

■ Other conditions can mimic the signs of dementia. The problems go when the basic cause is dealt with.

■ Too many drugs can leave an older person in a state of confusion and so can a poor diet and overuse of alcohol.

■ Ordinary illnesses can also lead to temporary confusion which can be mistaken for dementia. Brain tumours can press on the brain and cause behaviour changes and/or memory loss.

■ Depression can resemble dementia.

CHAPTER 3

The effects of dementia

· ·

This chapter looks at the effects that dementia has upon people's memories, feelings and behaviour. For people with dementia memory loss is a disability which makes everyday life difficult. Like everyone else, people with dementia may experience feelings of fear and anger, confusion and isolation; people with a damaged brain may actually have even more acute feelings than other people. 'Problem behaviour' may include wandering, accusations and challenging or embarrassing behaviour, but this should be put in perspective and seen as an attempt to communicate needs and feelings. Speech problems may include forgetting words, especially names, and nonsense chatter. The chapter concludes with a section on communicating more effectively with people with dementia.

· ·

Memory loss

People with dementia are in many ways like everybody else; they just have different problems from others. Whatever the losses, whatever the disability, we must remember that there is a unique person with the same humanity as the rest of us, the same type of history as many others, and similar needs to be loved and to love. If we concentrate too much on the losses that are inevitable in those who have dementia, we may miss the person and see only some unusual behaviour.

Many of the problems associated with dementia stem from the underlying problem concerning memory.

George had been living with his wife in Bristol for 35 years. He was asked at the bank to confirm his address, and astonished his wife by telling them that it was somewhere in Liverpool. That was where he lived when he was a boy long before he had moved to Bristol. What worried his wife most was that he didn't seem able to remember their present address at all.

'What did you have for lunch today?' asked **Meera**'s daughter when she visited the residential home for the first time after her mother had moved in. 'Oh, nothing at all', was Meera's reply. 'I didn't have anything yesterday either'. In fact, Meera had eaten well both at lunchtime and also the night before, but her damaged brain had erased the memory completely. The part of the brain that told her that she had eaten well was no longer working either, and she had no way of knowing that she had eaten and was really quite full.

Most of us are able to remember what we have forgotten. Sometimes we may put the oven on, prepare the chicken, and go out leaving the bird on the table. Half an hour later we suddenly remember what we have failed to do. Somebody with dementia would have no memory of needing to put the chicken in the oven at all. They might come home and wonder why there was a chicken on the kitchen table, and start asking how it got there. Any challenge about their failure to remember would probably be met with denial, arguments, accusations or tears.

Hoarding items with no rational explanation or purpose can also reflect the loss of recent memory. It is important to have enough toilet rolls, for example, in the house; so important that a person with dementia might buy a new stock on every visit to the shop. It may appear to be so vital as to be the only thing that is bought on each visit. A challenge to hoarding may bring angry defensive replies. The person with dementia may completely deny having anything to do with all the goods in the house.

Six different manifestations of memory loss are illustrated below:

Freda didn't recognise her husband when he came up to bed; she thought he was an intruder and screamed at him to get out. When he didn't do so, she picked up the phone and dialled for the police.

David had no idea of his son's name when he went on a visit. He knew that he was his son, but could not recall his name (or anybody else's name either).

Terry could never remember what he was going to do during the day. He would have little notes to tell him, but he often couldn't find them, so he had no idea what he was expected to be doing. His daughter found it all very annoying, especially when she went to a lot of trouble over his birthday lunch and he didn't turn up.

Ahmed kept on getting lost when he went for a walk. He would manage to get into town, but have no idea which road to take to get home again. Sometimes the police brought him home, which was an embarrassment to his wife, even though Ahmed seemed to find it quite enjoyable getting a lift in a police car.

Joy loved doing embroidery but as her dementia developed, she began to be less efficient, and eventually stopped doing it altogether.

Desmond was shown photos of his daughter's wedding. It had taken place only a few weeks before. Desmond had managed to walk down the aisle and give his precious daughter away. He couldn't understand the photo, didn't recognise himself, and, worst of all, denied that he had been there at all. He could remember his own wedding though.

Freda was unable to recognise faces, even the faces of people she knew well. Sacks tells of a man whose brain had been damaged in such a way that he was unable to recognise faces (among other things) but was still able to function well in his job as a music teacher (Sacks 1985). In his case the cause was not a dementia, but the symptoms are similar to those experienced by some people with dementia. For some there is a misidentification – for example a son may be thought of as a husband, who may have died long ago. This misidentification may be explained in part by the failure to understand that time has passed, that the husband has indeed died, and by the fact that the son (now middle-aged) may remind his mother of his father when he was at a similar age. Although the muddle can be understood, the emotional turmoil may be hard to cope with.

David's problem was a typical early sign of dementia. We all have difficulties with names of people we have just met for the first time. We may find it hard to remember the names of people we see on the news or read about in the papers; yet completely forgetting the names of members of our own family seems to be out of the question. People with dementia, however, may embarrass their families by their inability to remember such an important thing.

Terry's inability to get to lunch on his birthday was linked to his memory loss to do with forward planning. He could remember what had happened the day before, but the events of the future were something that his damaged mind was unable to cope with. Things like lists, a diary and a calendar helped him, but as time went by other skills disappeared and he was unable to remember where he had put the notes and the diary, and also forgot to look at them at the beginning of the day.

Ahmed had problems with his spatial memory. We all probably have a story of leaving the car in a car park, and then being totally unable to find it for several hours; but Ahmed was sometimes unable to retrace his footsteps. He would just be confused by all the choices in town and end up guessing the way back.

Joy had a memory problem to do with skills. The brain is full of the things that we have learned to do in the past. Some of them may be the skills we learned as a child, like washing or going to the toilet. Other skills will have been learned at a later stage. Some will be to do with our job, others to do with a hobby, or running a home. All of these are at risk with dementia.

Desmond's problem was to do with visual memory. Most of us can manage to conjure up pictures of important events in the past. Desmond could still manage to remember some of the events of his own earlier life, but the more recent events had already been erased from his memory bank.

Long-term, recent and short-term memory

Our memory of events can be divided into three basic categories:

Short-term describes the memory we need to remember a telephone number for the few seconds that it takes to dial the number. We may recall it well enough to dial it a second time if the first attempt goes wrong, but we usually forget it immediately afterwards as it becomes unnecessary information which we do not need to store in our memory bank.

Recent memory is the memory of what happened this morning, the route we took to get to work, or where the bus stop is. It is also the memory of yesterday's superb dinner with friends – we can picture the food, and remember some of the conversation.

Long-term memory is the store of things that have occurred in our life which for some reason or other we have retained, so that we can re-run them from time to time. Some of these long-term memory recalls may be a few months old, while others can go back to our early childhood.

Erasing the memory

If you imagine your memory as a videotape, it is very long-playing. At the beginning there are a few recordings of events of childhood. At the end there are the events of a few minutes ago. Most of the past has been erased because it is not needed, but there is footage of important happenings in our lives. People in advanced stages of dementia may be able to recall these events, but the disease may have erased most or all of what happened recently. That includes what happened five minutes ago; it includes what happened this morning, and last night, and last week, and a year ago. The long-term memories may be damaged too, and as the disease progresses they will increasingly be lost. As a result the erasing will carry on backwards down the years, erasing the memories of middle life, then the rest of adulthood, then the teen years, then the years of childhood. For a few there are no memories left at all.

With the disappearance of memory, the cognitive understanding vanishes too. Words fail, skills unravel, the personality may alter. However, nothing about dementia is straightforward: memory loss may not be total. What is forgotten today, may be suddenly remembered tomorrow, and then immediately forgotten again. It is now less like a video recording, and more like a torch with a poor connection. The torch refuses to work most of the time, but suddenly there is a beam of light in the darkness. This image describes the sudden flash of understanding, the sudden recall of something forgotten, which characterises many people with dementia.

Feelings

We should not forget that some people with dementia are quite happy. Others may experience emotions such as fear and frustration.

Fear and anger

Few have been able to describe what dementia is like, but Davis has described the experience like this:

> 'What was in my mind? Blackness and darkness of the worst kind. As soon as I let go of my concentration to try to fall asleep, there was nothing there. This vacuum was filled with terrifying blackness.'
> (Davis 1989)

Imagine for a moment what it might be like to step into the shoes of somebody with dementia – somebody whose memory played tricks on them and whose brain no longer produced the right words for the right occasion. Imagine finding yourself living in a strange house with no idea how you managed to get there. All the people are strangers; they tell you their names, but that means nothing to you. One or two claim to be your daughters, but you don't recognise them. They refuse to let you go home. They keep saying that your house has been sold, but you don't believe them. When you try to get out through the front door, they keep making you come back. They tell you that this is home, but it is nothing like any home you can remember. That one was in the country. This one seems to be in a suburban street, and you long for the days of old which you can see as clearly as if it was just yesterday. People come and talk to you, take you along the corridor and tell you to sit down at meals with total strangers.

Bik was walking down a corridor at a hospital. There were a couple of right-angle bends ahead of her, so she could only see a few metres in front of her. Her speed was dead slow. The nurse with her seemed to be pulling her along, although in fact she was only going a fraction faster. She said: 'I'm so frightened, I'm so frightened'. She had no idea where she was going. It would have been no use the nurse telling her that they had come along the corridor five minutes before. To her it was a totally strange place, with an unknown fate around the corner.

For the person with dementia no amount of reasoned explanation is going to deal with the fear of what is round the corner or the anger that they feel that their freedom seems to have been taken away from them. They may have even more acute feelings than other people. What is needed is loving acceptance and reassurance, and an acknowledgement of the fear that the person is experiencing.

Confusion

We are all confused at some time or another. So, when we say that people with dementia are suffering from confusion, we mean that their confusion is different from everyone else's.

First of all, it happens most of the time. The damage to the brain makes it difficult to interpret things correctly and so it is easy to make mistakes:

> **Fred** and his wife Mavis went on a holiday to Spain. On the first day Fred went down on his own to buy something at the shop in the foyer. When he came back he got out of the lift on the wrong floor and tried his key in someone else's door. He insisted that he was going in and even when the hotel management arrived, it took ten minutes to persuade him to go with them to the right floor. After that episode his wife felt that she could not let him out of her sight for the rest of the holiday.

Secondly, the confusion may be caused by the brain wrongly interpreting what is seen or heard:

> **Jean** was living in a care home. It had a lovely polished floor in the entrance area. Yet as Jean came down the stairs towards it, all she could see was the golden glow of the winter sun reflecting on the wood. It may have been beautiful, but to Jean it was scary and confusing, and she refused to set foot on it, however much the staff tried to persuade her. They thought she was being awkward, but what Jean saw, in her mind's eye, was a swimming pool filled with water, and she did not want to fall in and get herself soaked.

Thirdly, confusion can be caused by wrong identification:

> **Herbert**'s grandson looked to him just like his son. He kept on calling him by the wrong name, and could not understand who the middle-aged man

in the house was. When it was explained to him, it was only a matter of minutes before he was making the same mistake again.

Frustration and inadequacy

Learning can be a frustrating experience. Most of us have forgotten what it was like learning to tie our shoelaces or do up the buttons on a blouse, or write neatly, or ride a bike. It could be very frustrating when it all went wrong, and we were made to feel foolish. The same thing can happen when people with dementia are robbed of their skills.

Imagine for a moment that you are a DIY expert – you happily paint the house at the weekend, you wallpaper like a professional and you put in the new radiators. One day you know that you can't cope with the next job: you have actually forgotten how to get the screws into the wall. Frustration shortens your temper. So when you are asked why you have not got round to putting up the curtain rail, you say something fairly hostile and walk away as that is all you can think of doing about your crisis.

We may all feel daunted by a task we have to do. For someone with dementia, the feelings of inadequacy can lead to either aggression or withdrawal (the fight or flight syndrome). Losing skills and making mistakes leads naturally to a feeling of being inadequate. The feelings will be affected by the response of other people, at home or in the workplace. People may be laughed at for silly behaviour, be told off for doing the work wrongly or be treated as if they were little children and be talked to in a patronising tone of voice.

The illness itself causes some of the withdrawal, but some of it is linked to the way that people can be treated or even neglected. Withdrawal can have its own reward, especially in some care homes where the 'good' patient is the one who causes no bother, and conforms to what is expected by the staff. Dementia can make people become withdrawn or uncooperative and hostile, but good care and a focus on care for the individual can lessen that hostility, and help to soothe the frustrations and the inadequacies.

Abandonment and isolation

Roger had not had a holiday for years. His daughter had moved to Greece and he had never visited her there. A rest would be a good idea. His social worker was keen for him to have a break. She organised what she called 'respite' – an expensive stay for his wife **Helena** in a nursing home near the park. Helena even agreed to go. But Roger didn't feel too happy on the morning when he drove away from the home and got back to pack his suitcases for a solitary departure for the airport. As the plane took off from Gatwick, he wondered how his wife was getting on.

Helena spent her day and most of the night in a constant state of anxiety, wandering in the room and down the corridor. She kept on calling for Roger, and when he did not appear, she shouted to all who could hear that she had been abandoned. She was certain that he had gone off with another woman; and when the staff tried to tell her that the 'other woman' was in fact her daughter, she refused to believe a word of it.

A feeling of abandonment is common among those with dementia. It may happen in the family home with people all around or it might be triggered by the need to see parents again, to be cuddled by Mum, who may in the person's eyes have gone off and left them. The logical explanation, that Mum is dead, is unlikely to help. The world of people with dementia is likely to become more and more restricted as the illness takes hold. Withdrawing from what is a difficult and threatening world outside can lead to a very restricted existence. This can be especially the case when someone has lost a partner, but it can also be a lifestyle that develops as people get older; there is a loss of work-based activity, friends may be lost by death and moving away from the area, and it becomes safer and easier to stay at home.

The carer can take the brunt of the feelings of isolation (see Chapter 6).

Problem behaviour

Behind most of the 'problem' behaviour of people with dementia is the loss of the recent memory, or an inability to interpret the world around them correctly. They are trying to cope with a disability, but are not necessarily able to explain themselves in a way that the carer can understand.

When assessing a problem behaviour, the ABC approach can be very useful:

Antecedents. Is there anything in the individual's environment that triggers the behaviour? Examples might include being left alone, being insensitively handled, being unable to find the toilet, the disturbed behaviour of other residents, or being taken out of familiar surroundings. If such triggers can be identified and removed, this may solve the problem. Sometimes the trigger comes from within the individual: are they depressed, in pain, constipated, physically unwell, excessively sedated?

The **B**ehaviour itself. When considering a problem behaviour, it is always important to ask: for whom is it a problem? Is it causing the individual and others significant distress, or is it merely 'inappropriate' or inconvenient for family or care staff routines?

Consequences. All behaviours have consequences, and sometimes these can act to reward and reinforce the behaviour. For example, if shouting is the only means by which a resident can obtain contact with care staff, it is likely to persist. Problem behaviours are sometimes dismissed as 'attention-seeking', but it should be remembered that the desire for human contact is perfectly natural, whether or not one is suffering from dementia.

Lack of inhibition

We learn 'correct' behaviour as children. Dementia can damage these learned behaviours, so that a person may 'steal' from the supermarket or suddenly ask the girl at the check-out if she is married. It can make life rather embarrassing for a carer and puzzling for others:

Alrick worked for a care organisation. As part of his work it was agreed that he could take his client **Robert** out for lunch. It was one of those restaurants at the seaside with lots of tables placed close together and a waitress rushed off her feet. They had been waiting for a while, when the people at the next table were served. It was a trifle with a large red cherry on top – just what Robert wanted. He wasn't prepared to wait, and before he could be stopped, he had reached across and removed the cherry from the plate and popped it into his mouth.

The tact and inhibition centre of our brain is affected by dementia, so someone with dementia may say or do something which it is not normally acceptable for adults to do. Other examples might include:

- undressing in the High Street because it's suddenly got too hot;
- starting to sing *Nellie Dean* at full volume in the middle of a church service;
- following the zigzag patterns of the carpet like a two-year-old might do;
- insisting on talking to complete strangers on trains, when they obviously don't want to talk;
- going for a swim in a paddling pool and splashing all the children as if one of them; or
- trying to get into bed with the woman in the next room in the care home, even though she is frightened and calling for help.

A lack of inhibition can be coupled with a lack of perception and judgement. Sometimes this can appear to be a mark of what was once dismissively called 'second childhood'. Although it is a reminder of behaviour patterns from long ago, it in no way sums up the totality of their life. They are not children but people with damaged minds who sometimes behave spontaneously and who can find their environment difficult to cope with. In general the skills that have been learned earliest are the last to be damaged by dementia – skills which have become automatic are likely to be retained longer than ones which require judgement and understanding.

Loss of recognition skills/perception

People with dementia have problems interpreting the world that they see around them. Perception is affected and they may not see things as they really are and fail to recognise faces and places for example. It may make it impossible to get dressed without help if you cannot recognise the clothes: trousers may end up as unusual headgear and blouses be put on back to front.

People with dementia sometimes do not eat. They may not see food for what it is, and just leave it. This can be a major problem in hospital where the staff may just take the plate away with a comment about 'not being hungry today'. An inner sole may be taken out from a shoe, for example, and eaten because it looks like a piece of meat. Even where the food is recognised, the container may be totally unfamiliar, such as the tin foil containers that are used by some meals on wheels services.

Television can be another problem area. For most people with dementia the picture that they see is a confusing one. If they are watching a programme about, for example, starving children in Africa, the children may appear to be actually in the living room. Much of what is on the small screen is too fast for damaged brains to cope with. In care homes the set should only be switched on for a programme which is likely to be understood by residents.

Some of the problems of perception may be caused by other physical problems, such as poor eyesight or hearing, as well as by dementia. Spending all the time in artificial light or poor quality light may make it very difficult for those with damaged eyesight to see clearly what is around them. Glare on white walls or lots of shadows can give rise to hallucinations. Good design with pastel colours and lighting which provides for brightness without glare can do a lot to minimise the distortions that can arise (see pages 87–90 for more on building design issues).

Hearing difficulties may also lead to distorted understanding. The hearing impaired person needs to be able to see the person who is talking, and poor lighting once again does not help. People who wear hearing aids may hear extraneous noises all too well: in a new environment such as a care home they may misinterpret the sounds they hear. For example, a washing machine running in the kitchen may make them think that they are in a factory where they used to work.

Accusations

Ethel was unable to find her rings. She was certain that they had been beside her bed as usual yesterday, but today they were nowhere to be found. Her young grandson Aaron had come round in the evening, so she was sure that he must have them, and said so to his mother when she phoned. Aaron was upset that his gran should even think that he would take her rings. He knew enough about dementia to realise that she had probably put them somewhere safe and had forgotten all about it. He was right. They were eventually found in the kitchen drawer. 'I wonder how they got there', said Ethel.

Things can go missing in houses where there is someone with dementia. It may be a matter of trying to keep things safe or it may be bizarre behaviour which baffles everyone. Money can be flushed down the toilet, valuable documents thrown away, and photographs torn up and put in the waste-paper basket. When challenged, the person may deny any knowledge of the event, and proceed to blame someone else. Family and friends may be first to be accused, which can be especially hard, as false accusations undermine the trust and loyalty built up over the years.

Some accusations are, however, genuine. The difficulty is how to distinguish the true from the false:

> Alan used to go in every day to see his next-door neighbour **Sheelagh**. She could cope quite well with her dementia, but after a while things that were fairly new started to be replaced by older items. Sheelagh said that a man came in from time to time to do a swap, an old for new service. Alan thought that this was far-fetched and put it all down to the Alzheimer's disease which had just been diagnosed. He changed his mind, however, the Saturday morning he walked in on the 'transaction' and prevented a dealer from making off with a fairly new lawnmower.

People with dementia may need to be believed when they tell stories which are unusual. They can be at the mercy of those who might want to take advantage of their mental frailty.

Wandering

'Wandering' describes the pacing up and down, or the tendency to leave home to go for a walk and then be completely unable to find the way back again, which can be a feature of the behaviour of people with dementia. It can take the form of simply going off on their own in the middle of a shopping expedition or a trip to the seaside.

Of course it is not really wandering at all. It is a purposeful walk, but the purpose is kept hidden from the rest of us.

> Tracy took her Mum **Sandy** to the hairdresser's and said she would be back in an hour. Mum should wait there until she got back. An hour later Mum was nowhere to be found. She had told the staff she was going home

and had walked off in the wrong direction. The police found her late at night in the shopping centre and brought her home.

Nobody noticed **Walter** leave the residential home. He headed off into the country to try to find his old home in a nearby village. The shortcut he took led to a stream and he toppled in. It was several days before they found his body.

Annie kept on trying to get out at night. She would open the door at the end of the corridor that led to the fire escape. The alarm would sound and the staff would have to deal with other agitated people as well as Annie. All she wanted to do was to find her old home.

Gwen got a call from the police to say that they had found her sister **Sian** in Bristol. She had got there from her home in Brighton by train. The only trouble was that she had no idea where she was or how to get back home again.

Reasons for 'wandering' might include:

- a need for a walk
- to see the roses/ducks/children in the park
- to fetch the children from school
- to get the meal ready for the family
- to go home to Mum and Dad
- to find the real home
- to go to work
- to find somewhere better to spend the day

It may be impossible for a person with dementia to explain what they want. Even if they are able to explain, their explanation will probably sound ridiculous and they may not be listened to.

Frail and feeble, **Carmel** had to be guided everywhere in the house. She was quite likely to sit down in the wrong place, perhaps alongside the chair and land with a bump on the floor. One day the front door was open and Carmel was up from her chair, out of the door in a flash and off down the road, with her husband in pursuit. She was so fast that he could not catch up with her before she got to the main road at the bottom of the hill. Across she went without even a glance at the traffic. Fortunately there was nothing coming at that moment and she managed to cross safely. Coming back was a different matter, however, and it needed a friend's car to get them both up the hill and home.

Phyllis, aged 80, was no longer capable of walking more than a few steps without hanging on to the furniture. She lived in a nursing home a couple of miles away from her house which was now unoccupied. At about four o'clock one afternoon she was trying to get out of the front door after some visitors had left. Matron was trying to reason with her whilst keeping the door nearly closed. 'I've got to get home' Phyllis said repeatedly, 'I've got the whole family coming for a meal, and they'll be expecting me and now I've got to go and get the kettle on'. 'Now, wouldn't you rather have a nice cup of tea here in the lounge?' asked Matron. But that was no use. 'What would I be wanting a cup of tea for, when my family is waiting outside the house not able to get in?'

Phyllis might not have managed to get home with only one good leg. Some people with dementia, however, do have an ability to summon up immense strength and speed, and to make off into the distance. In the early stages of the illness people are often physically fit and need to have exercise.

One of the ways of ensuring that a person comes to no harm is to go with them. But sometimes carers are too busy to have the time, or in some cases are too frail themselves to manage to keep up.

Problems with routine tasks

Most routine jobs are in practice a series of activities. There are several stages involved in getting dressed for example, including choosing clothes suitable for the day (casual or formal, warm or cool); identifying the right clothes to put on first; identifying which hole the arms, legs and head go through; and using buttons and zips correctly. For many people with dementia the steps are too complicated to manage without help. Another example of a simple task is making a cup of tea. There are many steps involved in making tea properly. People with dementia are quite likely to return to a previous point in the process and, perhaps, keep on adding teabags.

The unfortunate result is that many people with dementia are unable to look after themselves properly if they live on their own. However, with help many people can cope with the basic tasks that they were previously able to do. They may need a helping hand, a reminder of the next step, and also a reminder that the gas or electricity needs to be turned off after the food has been cooked.

Driving

Driving is an example of an automatic skill. To drive a car requires co-ordination which at the beginning may take practice. A person who has been driving for 40 or 50 years can carry on using their driving skills without too much trouble in the early stage of the illness. However, there are other aspects of driving that may prove too difficult and lead to problems. Finding the way may be difficult; worse still is the perplexed driver whose dementia does not allow them to deal with the new one-way street system in town or the diversion because of an accident. Faced with these unexpected situations the driver may panic or spend time hesitating, and as a result become a danger to other road users.

The GP has the duty to inform the driving licence authorities that a patient is unfit to drive. The person with dementia also has this duty. If they want to continue to drive, they should request a medical examination from the DVLA.

Incontinence

Incontinence is not an early sign of dementia in most cases, but eventually incontinence of urine may develop and in later stages many people become incontinent of faeces as well. The reasons for this lie firstly in the failure of the brain to interpret correctly the signals from the bladder or bowels. Secondly, there is the problem of identification of the right place and the right receptacle to use. Unfortunately something like a waste-paper basket may be used as a toilet by somebody with dementia. Finding the right place requires a memory of the building. For some people that is not possible even in their own home. En-suite facilities in a care home may make the distance a short one, but they may not be recognised by older people who may expect the toilet to be down the corridor, or even down the garden.

Some of the people labelled as incontinent, therefore, have a problem connected with memory and awareness, or just with identifying the right door to go through. Labelling the door may help them, although that may depend on understanding symbols like a toilet bowl or being able to read. A coloured line leading to the toilet is another possibility. This solution may spoil the decor of the house or care home, however, and make it look more like an institution or a hospital. Way-finding assistance needs to be unobtrusive and yet easily picked out, as well as integral to the decor and even the design of the building (see pages 87–90).

People with dementia may need regular reminders of the need to go to the toilet. Reminders will help to minimise the amount of wet clothes and carpets, and also reduce the anxiety of those who are aware of their problems but have no secure memory of when they last went to the toilet. Regular toiletting according to the usual needs of the client will help. So too will an emphasis on continence, rather than on the failures which we describe as incontinence, as well as keeping an eye open for the signs of a need to empty the bladder (usually small movements showing that the person is getting uncomfortable). It is important to make sure that the person eats and drinks well. Good care of people with continence problems also includes record keeping. This should give the time that the person went to the toilet, and also an indication of fluid intake.

Self-expression

Changes in language

Derek does not say very much at all. He's in a world of his own today.

Tony is unclear because he can't find certain words any longer. He gets quite agitated about his difficulty. It must be frustrating to want to say something, but not have the words to do so.

Carlos is chattering away in Spanish. Nobody in the day centre understands what he is saying. He came to the UK 25 years ago, and used to be able to talk English, but he has forgotten it all (except on rare occasions) and is just left with Spanish now.

In the later stages of dementia there may be no communication through words. Even at an early stage, one of the signs of a person having difficulty may be in the use of language.

Chatter

For some people with dementia there is a constant chatter. It may take the form of a pouring out of language which makes no sense to the listener, talking to themselves, or bouts of shouting out or calling for help. It is important to try to bring comfort, to validate feelings, and not to say: 'It's no use calling for your mum; she's not here'.

The unfinished sentence

We all have moments when we forget our words; for people with dementia it can become the norm. The problem centres on nouns – ie words that are the names of objects and ideas – words like table, chair, bus, photograph, love, noise. Names of people and places – Albert, Irene, Gloucester Road and Birmingham – can also disappear, even if they are very important in a person's life. A whole story with no nouns is hard for a carer to understand. As time goes by, the sentences may get shorter until we are left with 'I' or 'We'.

Some people try to get round their problem by finding a long phrase to describe something, or use expressions like 'whatsit', 'thingummy', 'whatsitsname', or alternatively replace a word with another one in the same group ('train' instead of 'bus' for example).

Repeated questions

People with dementia often ask questions repeatedly, sometimes 10, 20, or 30 times in a space of minutes. This may be challenging for carers as they answer again and again and again but it can be worthwhile to try and understand what is behind the question.

It may seem as if the person with dementia is asking the same question on purpose just to annoy. But in fact the answer is forgotten immediately after it has been given. It is very insecure to be in the position of not knowing what is going on, and rather than the 'facts', the person may need validation (acknowledgement) of the feelings of loss or insecurity.

Poetic language

People with dementia may also make use of metaphor to express themselves; ie use a poetic language rather than a totally logical one. Killick has written about his experiences as a writer-in-residence at a nursing home where he has had the time to sit and listen to what people have to say.

They may use figures of speech that seem strange, but which express their deep-down feelings, as illustrated by the following lines a of a poem:

In the War I went around
And I saw nothing that wasn't
A waste of time and life.
The door opened to dust
And I thought it might be me tomorrow.
Now the evening is coming to a close for me.
You don't see your family
Much now; like a carrier bag
On your back, one way or another.
But you can't barge it or dish it –
All of it was everwell.
(Killick 1997a)

This poem presents a considered view of the past, the present and the future, complete with the image of the carrier bag denoting the transience of life. Killick succeeds in working with people who are apparently without speech. Just by sitting with them and being available for them, he finds, much to the surprise of relatives and staff, that some people with dementia may have a lot to say for themselves:

'The past, I think a lot about it. I'm thinking when ... I'm not saying ... I can't tell people things.'
(Killick 1997a)

Swearing

As there is damage to the area of the brain that deals with tact, modesty, and inhibition, there are often examples of people using language which shocks others. For example a person who has rarely, if ever, used four-letter words in conversation, now begins to use them frequently. There may be a general coarsening of language with jokes told that would not have been told previously.

This can be difficult for families and friends to cope with, and especially difficult when it takes place in public. Some people may also be aggressive in their speech. The bad or aggressive language may suggest a change in personality, or it may be the emergence of aspects of personality that have been hidden. A smile, a little reassurance, and above all a refusal to be confrontational, are all ways of helping to get the person back on an even keel.

People from other countries and cultures

People whose English language skills have been learned in later life are likely to lose these skills before their first language skills. One example of the problem is given in Heywood's book *Caring for Maria* (1994). Maria was his upstairs neighbour, a friend of many years, who had come to Britain in 1949. At an early stage of Maria's dementia, Heywood says:

> 'This German language business with her confused mind is so strange. For example, when I ask if *leben* means 'to live', she just repeats it. She then goes off into some sort of roundabout explanation (in German), not understanding that all I want is a simple yes or no. Then she says I'm an idiot. She doesn't seem to grasp that German isn't English, or that English isn't German when I speak it.'
> (Heywood 1994)

Maria had got to a point where she did not recognise the difference between the languages she was using, and just expected Heywood to be able to understand her. It may be necessary for native speakers and others with foreign language skills to be invited in to help to communicate with people like Maria as well as people who have never learned English and who will only be able to communicate in their native language.

Communicating with people with dementia

Busy carers can sometimes fail to communicate effectively with the people they are looking after. It can be easy to forget basic principles of communication and give messages that are uncaring or overbearing.

Some suggestions for improving communication include:

1 Make sure that the person realises that you are trying to talk to them. Face them. If they are sitting down, try to be on the same level; perhaps you can sit down alongside them. Use gentle touch to show that you want to communicate, and also to have a calming effect. Try to maintain eye contact as you speak.

2 Use short sentences and simple, straightforward ideas. Say, for example, 'We're going out to the shops'. Don't then add, 'And then we'll visit Jane, and if she's in, we'll take the children for a walk round the park.'

3 Allow time for a reply and try to hide your impatience. Silence may be needed for somebody with dementia to respond.

4 You can communicate in other ways than by words. Touch may be a first indicator that you want to say something. It can reassure, and show love and warm feelings. Body language and gestures may give meaning when words no longer have any meaning. It is therefore important to know what signals you are sending out. For example, most people look cross when they have their arms folded. Smiling can reassure.

5 Don't underestimate the power of tone. The message may be in words, but the tone may reveal kindness or impatience. The same words can be said in perhaps half a dozen different ways, and give a range of messages beyond the intention of the speaker. For example, a question like 'Are you ready now?' can sound like an accusation; a different tone and stress pattern can turn it into something gentle and unthreatening.

6 As some people with dementia have problems with recognising family and friends, it may be necessary to say who you are and where the person is living (see pages 95–96 on Reality Orientation).

Key points

■ As people with dementia are unable to interpret events around them, they may experience a range of feelings such as anger, fear, confusion and isolation.

■ People may suffer from different types of memory loss, for example an inability to recognise faces. Recent memory is affected rather than long-term memory.

■ Behaviour which can be seen as a problem by others includes: 'wandering'; incontinence; accusations; and difficulties with interpreting what is happening and with routine tasks.

■ A better understanding of what the person is trying to do or say, will make for better care.

■ Problems with speech may include: forgetting words (nouns first of all); not finishing sentences; swearing; or chatter which appears to make no sense.

■ People from other countries may lose their English language skills first.

■ When talking to someone with dementia, use short sentences and simple ideas as well as the correct tone and body language.

CHAPTER 4

Care for people with dementia

Community care

● ●

It can be difficult to get a diagnosis of dementia as there may be no clinical signs, although there are tests which can show the changes in the brain. The first part of this chapter explains that GPs can refer people to a specialist for further tests and for scans. After a diagnosis most people have no idea what support services are available to them and their families. This section describes: possible routes that doctors can use to enable people to gain access to suitable services; ways in which to help people stay in their own homes; and the problems that they may encounter in using services in the community.

● ●

Diagnosis

Diagnosis of dementia is not straightforward. A doctor may believe that the condition is merely a matter of normal ageing or that the patient is suffering from some form of mental illness, such as depression. As a result there is a wide range of categorisation which is to be found even today. Terms such as 'softening of the brain' are no longer used, but instead we have terms like 'confusion' and 'memory loss', which are merely descriptions of problems that patients may be having but which are unacceptable as a diagnosis.

Dementia does not have the sort of tell-tale signs which can give a speedy and accurate diagnosis. Lovestone's research (see page 3) indicates the complexities of this area of medicine. In the early stages of Alzheimer's disease the patient gives every sign of normality in the surgery and can even appear to be in vigorous good health. Meanwhile the carer may be looking strained and anxious, unable to sleep properly because of the behaviour of their partner or parent; they may even end up being diagnosed with stress.

Dorothy lived with her sister **Bessie**. Bessie suffered from heart trouble as well as having many of the symptoms of dementia. The GP was only interested in the heart condition. When Dorothy asked him what could be done about her sister's unusual behaviour and poor memory, he just shrugged his shoulders and indicated that there was nothing he could do. As far as he was concerned Alzheimer's was a rare condition of younger people, whilst in older people it was senile dementia. No referral, therefore no diagnosis.

Carers faced with a situation like Dorothy's should insist on a referral. If they are not listened to, further help and advice can be obtained from the Alzheimer's Society – see page 121 for the address.

Getting a diagnosis

The first port of call is the General Practitioner (GP). In general, patients and their families are able to give the doctor enough information for a case history to be written up – in cases of dementia, however, patients alone can be unreliable. They may minimise the problems or even deny that there is anything the matter. They may for example say that they are able to do their own shopping, whilst in reality it is always done by a member of the family. A person may claim to cook meals every day, but in practice be incapable of using the oven or even boiling a kettle.

The carer may be the chief source of information. They may tell the doctor or nurse how things really are, listing the things that their relative is no longer able to do, and describing strange behaviours, such as wandering off down the road and not being able to find the way back. It can be hard for the GP to decide who to listen to when there may be a history of friction and the carer may appear to be stressed and unreasonable.

A home visit is far better than any trip to the surgery for anyone with dementia, and should be offered even for the first consultation if there is any hint that dementia is suspected. At home the person can be seen in their own environment. There may be mess and muddle; clues concerning behaviour patterns; and photographs and other material which may help the GP or practice nurse to probe into memory lapses. It may be possible for the GP to get the patient to do some activity that they claim to be able to do regularly, such as making a cup of tea.

Doctors and their receptionists may complain that they do not have the time to make such visits to people who are fit enough to make the journey to the surgery, but physical fitness should not be the sole criterion. More important is whether the existence of a condition such as dementia is going to be discovered by requiring patients to make a journey which may prove a waste of time if they are uncooperative. One possibility is for a Community Psychiatric Nurse (CPN) to make the visit as they are trained to deal with a whole range of mental conditions including dementia.

Asking questions to test for possible dementia

The consultation will probably by now have taken over the five or seven minutes of time that is normally allocated in the surgery. The GP should, however, make the time to ask the ten questions which form the abbreviated Mini-Mental State Examination (MMSE). These are questions which most people would be able to answer without any problem at all – things such as the day of the week, where they live etc. A score of lower than six out of ten can be followed up by the full MMSE, which involves tests of a wider nature. It includes some simple calculation, and the copying of a simple diagram. A score of less than 24 out of 30 indicates that further tests are needed. However, it is clearly of no use in determining dementia in someone with learning difficulties or someone who cannot read or write. Similarly, the questions should be culturally appropriate. The person's history should be available to the GP, and the carer can give important information about the capabilities of their relative. Indeed, it may be a catastrophic decline in the skills of their relative which has brought them to the surgery in the first place.

Other possible diagnoses

It is important at this stage for alternative causes of the dementia condition to be explored. There is a range of conditions which may be quite rare, but which could be the explanation for the confusion or the memory loss. Some of these can be cured or at least controlled (see pages 26–31). The following tests will enable other conditions (such as hyperthyroidism and vitamin deficiency) to be eliminated:

- a full blood count
- vitamin B12
- liver and thyroid function
- urea and electrolysis
- calcium and glucose

Referral to a specialist

Many GPs can make a diagnosis without the need for a referral. As the number of people in the very old category is increasing, and with it the number of cases of dementia, specialists' caseloads are increasing and it may be felt that no great purpose would be served in making a referral anyway. Specialist referral will be needed, however, if a patient might benefit from one of the drugs for Alzheimer's disease and these are only available locally from specialist services. Moreover, specialists have both expertise and equipment that GPs do not have and can help families get access to the community services that they need.

Under 65

Below the age of 65 a person with dementia will usually be pointed in one of two directions – neurologists or psychiatrists. Neurologists will be able to order scans of the brain to see if there are any abnormalities which might explain the condition. They might, for example, find that the dementia is caused by a brain tumour, which may be operable.

Psychiatrists are more likely to look for a mental illness. There will be a closer look at behaviour, and the patient might be admitted to the psychiatric ward at the local hospital along with others who might be suffering from a range of psychiatric illnesses. Here the staff are likely to spend time observing. Other patients will be suffering from conditions such as depression, schizophrenia, or bi-polar (manic depressive) mental illness. The younger the person, the more likely that the condition will be seen as psychiatric; dementia is unlikely to be suspected, and a correct diagnosis may therefore be difficult to make.

In some areas there are specialist 'memory clinics' that are equipped to provide a detailed diagnostic assessment of mild and questionable cases. There is usually no age barrier, and many clinics have a particular interest in early onset dementia.

Over 65

Responsibility for people over 65 lies with old age psychiatrists (sometimes known as 'psycho-geriatricians') although there may still be some referrals to psychiatrists or neurologists (in some areas, old age psychiatrists also deal with younger people with dementia). In areas which have been able to set up suitable services, they may have a day hospital as a base, and be able to see patients for much longer than a few minutes. Alternatively, there may be a specialist unit which has similar facilities, but which can also offer respite (holiday) care. In some parts of the UK these units are run jointly by the health authority and social services. Old age psychiatrists are responsible for the full range of mental health of older people, including depression and schizophrenia, but with the emphasis on the growing area of dementing illnesses. It can be all too easy for dementia to be diagnosed when the patient is suffering from a mental illness like depression; the exact opposite of what is likely to occur with people of a younger age.

More tests

As memory loss does not only affect general knowledge or the ability to calculate, the specialist may also test other skill areas, such as language skills and practical skills. These tests are particularly important when somebody is suffering from frontal lobe (fronto-temporal) dementia, as for them cognitive understanding and general knowledge can be relatively unaffected by the illness.

Language tests

Language tests involve word links. For example, a person might be asked to name all the things they can think of beginning with a particular letter. People with dementia are likely to be able to remember only two or three. Groups of words may also prove difficult, such as words to do with sport or transport. The memory can be tested with groups of words which are given with a request for them to be repeated immediately. Then they can be requested a second time a few minutes later. People with dementia are likely to have forgotten the words after several minutes, while some may have a complete inability to recall any immediately after having heard them.

Practical tests

Practical tests require a person to show how to use or do something. Such a test can be achieved by a simple request to, for example, use a comb or a pen. The tester could then show a person how to do an activity and ask them to repeat it. This requires use of the frontal lobes which direct operations in the brain and are in charge of the 'how to' or management part of the brain. Failure here is again especially prevalent in Pick's Disease, but it is also a feature of other dementias.

One commonly used test for damage to the brain is the copying of a clock face; for example asking the patient to draw a clock face showing a particular time. Different patients will interpret the request in a range of different ways. Some will start the activity and then forget what they are supposed to be doing. As a result they may end up with a clock showing 30 hours. Others are liable to leave out some numbers, failing to keep to a sequence that they would previously have followed automatically. The standard of circle for the clock will also vary. Finally, there may be someone who interprets the job more literally than most: they draw the clock and put in a mouth, a nose and two eyes. Some of this reveals damage which puts the sufferer back to a developmental level of a child in nursery school, adding weight to the theory that people with dementia lose faculties and skills in roughly the same order that they acquired them when they were small children.

Scans

Scans enable doctors to see what is happening inside the brain. In theory it should be easy to see the damage that is done by the various dementias, just as it is possible for X-rays to show a broken arm or the presence of tuberculosis.

CT (Computed Tomography)

The first scan became available in 1974. A CT scan is able to show a cross-section of the brain, and to confirm the loss of neurones which was identified by Alzheimer as one of the signs of dementia at post-mortem. Unfortunately, the same shrinkage is also visible in the scans of some older people who do not have any sign of dementia. More useful is a series of scans taken at intervals of several months as these show the pro-gressive shrinking of the brain. CT scans have proved to be more useful as a diagnostic tool when the temporal lobes are examined rather than a cross-section of the whole brain.

MRI (Magnetic Resonance Imaging)

CT scans are cheaper than the MRI scans which followed them. However, MRI scans are more versatile and give a better detail of the outlines of the structures of the brain.

SPET (Single-Photon Emission Tomography)

SPET measures the blood flow in the brain. Reduced flow in a particular area is linked to a decline in the ability of the brain to undertake tasks – for example, memory loss is linked to a reduced flow of blood in the temporal lobes.

PET (Positron Emission Tomography)

PET is a three-dimensional tool which enables functional changes in the brain to be seen, such as blood flow and glucose utilisation. Some brain dysfunction can even be detected before actual cell loss has taken place. This clearly gives it a great advantage over CT and MRI which show up actual rather than future cell loss. However, PET is very expensive and the equipment is only available in a few academic centres in the UK.

Scans can be useful tools for doctors in making a diagnosis, and vital for researchers in their quest for better understanding of disease, but they may not prove easy to administer with people whose brains have been damaged by dementia. Any examination by a doctor may cause problems, even the journey to the surgery; so it is quite likely that being placed in a machine and told to lie still may cause someone with Alzheimer's or Pick's Disease a great deal of anxiety. Anxiety leads very quickly to behaviour which would make it difficult to continue the scan.

Right to know a diagnosis

If a scan has been carried out, the question arises as to who should be told the diagnosis – whether it is the carer or the person with dementia who is the client.

> Harry was certain that his wife **Audrey** would get upset if she knew that she had Alzheimer's disease. She could accept that she had some memory problems, and that her brain was no longer as good as it was, but she was never told that she had an illness with a name, as Harry made quite sure that friends and family never mentioned the words 'Alzheimer's' or 'dementia' to her. All his newsletters from the Alzheimer's Society were delivered to a friend's house across the road, and when he went to his carers' meeting, he never let her know exactly where he was going. He said he was trying to protect her, but some of the family felt that it made him secretive and gave an opportunity for his wife to make accusations about him.

This situation is very similar to what used to happen in the diagnosis of cancer a generation ago. The fear of a dreaded illness was such that the family tried to ensure that their loved one was kept in ignorance of the real facts. This conspiracy between the medical team, the family and friends resulted in an invisible barrier, a lack of frankness, developing between them and the person with the illness.

In the past, people with Alzheimer's and other dementias were referred to specialists at a relatively late stage and were therefore perhaps not able to understand what was being said about them and their illness. Earlier referral has, however, resulted in people being told the bad news at a relatively early stage in the illness. That includes younger men and women who are still sometimes able to hold down a job, and who have every wish to be kept informed about what is happening to them. When the family and doctors keep the diagnosis to themselves, it is usually intended to avoid causing unnecessary suffering, but it takes away from the person with dementia the possibility of putting their affairs in order, organising power of attorney and making decisions about the future with the family. It may be a frightening prospect, but it can also be something which can be shared, and even grieved over together.

After a diagnosis

To be told that you have Alzheimer's disease will be a shock, but it can be an even greater shock for the carer. To begin with, the news may not fully register and the implications may take time to sink in.

> Olive was told by the specialist that her husband **Rodney** was suffering from dementia and that there was nothing that could be done. She had no idea how the illness would develop nor how she could get support. It was only when she saw an article in a magazine that she realised where she could get some help from.

> Gustave's family doctor asked him to come to the surgery half an hour before the usual opening time and gave him time and space to ask questions about how he could care for his wife **Bridget.** Gustave really appreciated being given a few key phone numbers to ring. It made all the difference having people who would give him the information that he needed and listen to him when he was feeling particularly stressed.

> **Richard** was able to understand what the doctor told him. When the initial shock had passed, he felt happy that he was able to take charge of his life. He could organise his early retirement, and had the opportunity of travelling to Australia to see his daughter. He could also make sure that the family finances were in order. Above all he was able to talk to his wife Emily about the situation and together they could plan for his nursing care.

After a diagnosis has been given, it is important that there are opportunities for counselling and for receiving information from a professional, such as a social worker or a nurse. Admiral Nurses are employed in some areas of London. They have specialist knowledge of dementia and can be contacted through the Dementia Relief Trust (address on page 124). The

Alzheimer's Society (see page 121) has a helpline and branches in most parts of the country. Many branches have carers' meetings and local helplines as part of their activities.

The support system

Ideally a person with dementia should stay in the security of their own home for as long as possible. For that to happen they need a considerable amount of support from a range of services. What happens in practice varies from person to person, even in areas where the services are good.

Most services are accessed via the local social services department. The carer, a family member, a neighbour or somebody from a voluntary organisation, such as Age Concern or the Alzheimer's Society, can phone and ask to speak to the duty officer. Social services must then make an assessment of the needs of the person with dementia and also those of the carer. It is intended that from April 2001 a carer can ask for an assessment even if the person they care for refuses one, perhaps because they have not accepted that they have an illness.

A needs assessment should result in everyone agreeing a care plan. This may involve a home care assistant, who might help with getting somebody up in the morning or to bed at night. It might give access to a day centre and the meals on wheels service. The social worker also assesses whether there is a need for residential or nursing home care. Carers can ask for a needs assessment for themselves. It is intended that from April 2001 carers can receive services in their own right; emphasis has been placed on the need for carers to have a break.

Local authority decisions on eligibility for services, on what services will be provided, and on how much will be charged for them, can be challenged; if carers feel that decisions are wrong, they are fully entitled to appeal against them.

> Age Concern Factsheet 41 *Local Authority Assessments for Community Care Services* gives further information about the assessments. See page 132 for details of how to obtain Age Concern factsheets.

Other community care staff who might become involved include occupational therapists, who are responsible for helping people to cope with the ordinary day-to-day skills of life (for example how to use a kettle safely) and for arranging for any aids and adaptations to the home which may be required. Nurses may be needed to deal with other conditions – for example, dementia is often linked to falls; people with dementia may be prone to more infections than others if they are not looking after their health very well; and they may need help in staying continent.

Services in the community

Day centres

For those with dementia a day centre is a place where they can meet others, have a midday meal, and engage in a range of activities. For the carer it offers a few hours of peace and quiet from the hectic round of a non-stop day and sometimes a disturbed night as well. Good day centres are modern and spacious, in refurbished and specially designed buildings, with expert staff to look after the clients. Ideally there is freedom to move about inside the building with a garden outside which is enclosed and safe. In one day centre in East Sussex a volunteer receptionist has a desk at the front door, and so can notice somebody leaving the building; the staff also keep an eye open for those who might want to go for a walk and often accompany them.

This centre is open some evenings and at weekends, but take-up is not always as good as the staff would want, perhaps because of the charges that are made. Transport can be a problem too. Volunteer drivers are often needed because of the costs involved. At this Sussex day centre the problem has to a large extent been solved by the use of local taxis whose drivers seem expert in the care of the people who attend the centre.

Respite and emergency care

All carers need time off. Day centres and day hospitals provide regular short breaks from the task of caring, and longer periods of respite can be arranged by admitting the person with dementia for one or two weeks on a regular basis to a specially designated hospital 'respite care' bed.

Respite care is also necessary to cope with emergencies in the home. A carer may fall ill, or someone else in the family may have an accident or an operation, and the carer suddenly has a double responsibility. A respite care bed for a week or two may enable the carer to cope. The problem with sudden or unexpected admissions to respite care is that the person with dementia is unlikely to understand what the emergency is. They may have no conception of anyone else's needs, and only see the move in terms of being abandoned by the carer. Feeling isolated, they are prone to illness and accident.

> Winifred had to go into hospital suddenly to have an operation. The usual respite care centre was unable to find a bed at short notice, and Winifred's husband **Roland** had to be admitted to another one. Within days he had picked up one of the winter viruses, which developed into a major chest infection followed by pneumonia. Although Winifred made good progress herself, it was only fast enough for her to get to her husband's funeral. Years of patient caring had come to an end without her being able to nurse her husband at the end of his life.

Winifred might have reproached herself for her 'failure' to care; however, the only alternative might have been the costly, and equally disruptive, one of carers looking after him at home.

Care in the person's own home

Day centres and respite care are two examples of services which might be available in the community, but it is also necessary to provide a package of care which will give practical and emotional help within the person's own home. For some it can be an expensive business, costing just as much as a stay in a nursing home (charges for local authority services will, however, be limited to what is considered a 'reasonable' amount; forthcoming government guidance will seek to minimise regional variations in charges).

Crossroads

The Crossroads Care Attendant scheme operates in over 100 different parts of the UK (the address of the national office is given on page 124). The scheme is funded through a mixture of grants from bodies like social services, and donations from the public. The carer is encouraged to make a donation, but there is no actual charge (in most schemes). Care may, however, be available for no more than a couple of hours once a week.

Although it only gives the carer the time to go to the supermarket to do the week's shopping, that may seem like a treat to a carer who never gets outside the front door. The staff come with an understanding of the needs of a range of people with special needs, including those who have some form of dementia. There are similar organisations throughout the UK, funded and encouraged through local agencies, which can be contacted via social services or the Alzheimer's Society.

Independent care providers

Over the last few years there has been a large rise in the number of independent (private) care providers, often contracted through social services. They have largely taken the place of the home help service run directly by social services. Age Concern Factsheet 6 *Finding Help at Home* (see page 132) provides information on how to access them. Some workers in this sector are highly trained and capable of nursing people recovering from a serious operation or in a terminal stage of their illness. At the other end of the scale there are many unqualified and inexperienced people who do tasks for which they may have had no training whatsoever. However, a well-qualified nurse may not have expertise in working with people with dementia, whilst an 18-year-old on a working holiday may have enough empathy and understanding of people to cope quite easily with a person with dementia.

> **Kate** lives on her own in a superb flat overlooking beautiful scenery. She is no longer really mobile. She is able to talk but has very poor memory. She is unable to do much for herself, but eats well, and is still fairly fit despite her dementia and inability to walk far. Her carer is a friend, Louise, who lives in a nearby flat. There is no family near enough to take any part in Kate's care. So Louise has taken over and made major decisions. She is a dynamic organiser, active and knowledgeable. She visits every day, but knows that at her own advanced age she cannot take over the full-time care of her friend. She has engaged a company to provide live-in care at a reasonable price. At present that means two young sisters from Australia. She provides them with a list of instructions and sees that they are carried out. Fortunately she is not only demanding but also very friendly and encouraging. There is a range of literature available in the flat about dementia, as she knows that

the girls (and most of the other staff) have no training. Kate is alert and talkative. She looks forward to going out with the girls around the district after lunch. The present arrangements are probably working well.

The best care providers try to arrange planned care, matching the needs of the client and the skills and experience of the care worker. In the case of dementia care that means that care workers must have an understanding of dementia before they start work in someone's home. Ideally:

- Staff will have been trained in basic dementia awareness.
- If not already trained, the staff must be ready to learn from the carer and other sources about the nature of dementia.
- Staff must be prepared to learn the particular needs of the person they are looking after.
- Staff need to know or discover which activities are suitable.
- Staff should be totally honest. Vetting procedures need to be rigorous.

Friends and neighbours

Friends and neighbours are a vital part of the support network. They may be able to take someone out for the afternoon, or come in and sit for a while so that the carer can get out and have time alone. A former workmate may be able to chat about the memories of the past. A friend might be able to come in and do something practical like cooking or gardening. The church, mosque or synagogue authorities could make sure that regular visits are made to those they know about.

Such visits are vital so that a carer can be relieved of duties for a while. They are also needed when the person with dementia lives alone. Some areas have volunteer visitors organised through the local volunteer bureau. Some older pupils do community service as part of personal and social education at school or college. Where a residential home is close to a school, there can be opportunities for visits by the choir for example. Reminiscence work (see pages 96–97) could be part of the history curriculum. Older people are primary sources of information and may be able to tell accurate stories of life in the past even when the activities of today and yesterday are quickly out of their minds.

Problems in using community services

People who work in the community are often not ready to deal with the problems that can be posed by someone with dementia. In a supermarket or on a bus it is perhaps not surprising that staff are unprepared, but it is far less understandable when staff working in the caring professions do not understand or make allowances either.

The doctor's surgery

People with dementia rarely go to the doctor's, especially in the earlier stages of the illness. Once there, in order to get a flu jab for example, there is the problem of the ten minutes or more in the goldfish bowl of the waiting room. There are toys for the children and magazines for the adults but probably nothing to occupy or distract someone with dementia. Loud comments or embarrassing questions may make the carer feel that ten minutes is a lifetime.

The receptionist, practice manager and other staff can help by identifying the patients who might be suffering from dementia and who might be confused enough to have problems while they are waiting. We have seen that, because of a general lack of proper diagnosis, surgeries may not know which patients suffer from dementia. Once this understanding has been achieved, a strategy to ensure a smooth and uneventful visit to the surgery might involve arranging an appointment at the beginning of surgery hours, when there is little likelihood of the doctor running late and keeping the patient waiting. Another possibility is a home visit, which could be done by the practice nurse. It has the benefit of avoiding the stress of a journey to the surgery and also means that the person can be seen in their normal environment.

The dentist

The problems of waiting are the same at the dentist's as they are at the doctor's. Finding a dentist who keeps to time throughout the day is important for the carer of someone with dementia. Both dentist and receptionist need to be made aware of the dementia condition of the patient so that they can be extremely careful to make the atmosphere even calmer than usual. A different house or building is enough to confuse someone with dementia; a dentist's chair and the noise of a drill may cause a panic reaction in someone unable to work out what is going on. As with the doctor, a home visit, where possible, may be preferable.

Hospital – Accident & Emergency

A long wait in Accident & Emergency (A&E) as a non-emergency case can be very problematic for someone who does not understand why they have to wait, or even why they have to be there in the first place. Staff in A&E, particularly the triage nurse (the nurse who sees the patient on arrival at A&E and who makes a decision about the urgency of the accident or illness), should be on the lookout for the word 'dementia', said by the carer, or for behaviour which might look like the effects of dementia. Then, if possible, the patient should be given priority for the benefit of both patient and staff.

Admission to hospital

Being admitted to hospital can be a frightening experience for anybody; for those with dementia there can be a feeling that they have been abandoned by their carer. Medical and domestic staff may not necessarily understand the problems of having someone with dementia in their ward. Information about the condition may be forgotten because the focus of the staff's attention will be the illness or the accident that has brought the person to the hospital, and not the underlying dementia.

Hospital staff need to be aware that people with dementia may be unable to understand what is going on in the ward. They may have a completely different perception of life in hospital and only make sense of it in the light of events in their past. For example there are still older people who have vivid memories of life in prisoner-of-war camps in the Second World War.

A dementia patient in a ward may not be able to:

- communicate needs
- remember instructions
- recognise food and drink
- eat and drink before the tray is removed

They may:

- try to get out of bed when they have been told to stay there
- try to leave the building to go home or to find their carer, even if attached to a drip or catheter
- be aggressive and uncooperative in dealings with the staff
- shout out and disturb others in the ward
- become acutely confused (people with dementia are particularly vulnerable to developing delirium if they are physically ill)

However harassed staff are, it is essential to realise that it is necessary to find the time to talk quietly and calmly to the person. On an understaffed, hectic surgical ward this may be difficult to do, as staff under pressure may only see an awkward patient whom they don't understand and don't have the time and resources to cope with. There may also be the feeling that such patients should not be on a general ward and that ordinary nursing and care staff are not adequately trained to deal with them. The information about person-centred care later in this chapter applies here (pages 78–92).

People with dementia may not be able to look after themselves properly in the recovery stage. They may not, for example, understand why there are tubes in place and so try to remove them, or they may not be able to feed themselves even if they do so normally at home. They may not be able to get to the toilet and back to their bed unaided. If left in the toilet, they may try to get out and fall over. On the other hand, over-protection may reduce independence. It may be easier and less time-consuming to take the person to the toilet in a wheelchair, but mobility needs to be maintained. In extreme cases, the final state of the patient at the point of discharge is one of complete disorientation and dependency.

The Care Passport

Identifying the person with dementia is one of the main difficulties for hospital staff. One solution, which has been trialled in Eastbourne and the Wealden area of East Sussex, is the 'Care Passport' scheme. This is an A5 document which is intended to supplement the normal notes, and to be placed where all staff can easily read it. It contains very simple information about the patients such as:

- My wife is unable to feed herself without help.
- My husband is unable to ask to go to the toilet.
- My mother cannot pass on any information.

It is important that both staff and carers realise that the passport must not be put among the rest of the patient's notes where it will stay out of sight as far as most of the staff are concerned. Some nursing staff object to its use because it breaks confidentiality. It does, however, give information to all staff, including the domestic staff, and is readily accessible. Others may object that it singles out a particular patient or group of patients and as a result labels them. Nonetheless it is a low-key system of highlighting to staff the fact that people with dementia require special care. The scheme makes it more likely that there will be high standards of care for this group of clients and lessens the risk of malnutrition and dehydration. Encouraging its use will make it easier for all staff to do their job efficiently and without additional stress. It also enables the carer to feel confident that their relative will be looked after well throughout their stay in hospital.

Further information about the Care Passport scheme is available from the area office of Care for the Carers – see page 123 for the address.

Sheltered housing

Living in a warden-controlled flat or bungalow can be an ideal way of staying independent whilst also having someone who can easily be called upon in an emergency. However, whilst it may be quite acceptable to look after someone who has flu for a fortnight, it is not part of a warden's duties to care for a person who is suffering from dementia. There may be conflicts between residents, as others may feel that it is wrong for them to have to live in the same place as people who perhaps seem to threaten their security and well-being. Some wardens feel that a sheltered home should be as much home as any other home might be and that people should not be removed because they are beginning to behave in a way which upsets some of the other residents. It might be unwise for sheltered housing schemes to offer leases to people who are clearly suffering from dementia already, but it is another matter entirely to force someone to leave their home because of problems that develop after they have taken up residence.

However, the warden cannot be expected to do the work of a family carer and be responsible for the general welfare of other people as well. Residents with dementia need social and health services support in just the same way that they would if they were living on their own. Other residents can also be encouraged to offer support in the same way that people are looked after unofficially by neighbours and friends.

Key points

- Dementia can sometimes be difficult to diagnose as there are no physical signs which point directly to it.

- GPs can refer to a specialist after taking a brief history from the patient and the carer, and a short test of mental skills.

- At age 65 people are referred to the psycho-geriatric service (old age psychiatrists).

- Specialists have a wider range of cognitive tests as well as the benefit of scans.

- The diagnosis of dementia is still often withheld from people so as not to upset them. There is a need to share the diagnosis with them.

- People staying in their own homes need a package of care which may involve independent care providers, day centres or a Crossroads Care Attendant scheme.

- People can encounter problems waiting at the doctor's or dentist's or the hospital.

- In-patients with dementia may be helped through the Care Passport scheme, which enables staff to identify those who may be unable to communicate or feed themselves.

- Wardens of sheltered housing schemes need support if they have a resident with dementia.

Long-stay care

The 1980s saw the closure of the old geriatric hospitals and an increase in the number of private residential and nursing homes. This section describes the different types of care homes, looks at the issue of paying for long-term care, and discusses the pros and cons of long-stay care compared to care in the community.

Types of care homes

The old geriatric hospitals were huge and found in every town. Today, beds in such institutions are few in number.

Most towns also had local authority homes, which were known as 'Part Three Homes'. Like the geriatric hospitals, they accommodated people with dementia, but they were not designed for them. The major difference for the customer was that you paid the local authority for a room there, but a bed in a hospital was free (like the rest of the National Health Service). In place of all these today there is firstly the assessment unit, then the day centre and the respite care unit, or long-stay care in a nursing home or residential home.

Nursing homes offer nursing care after an operation or during a serious illness. They are also home to people who have a long-term health problem, or who need a considerable amount of nursing care. Nursing homes must have a Registered General Nurse (RGN) on duty at all times. Their registration and inspection is the responsibility of the local health authority.

Residential homes do not offer nursing care, although they will look after residents who are ill for a short period of time. There is no need for a nurse to be on duty, as residents are not expected to need nursing care. They may need help with dressing and eating, or they may be disorientated, but they do not need the same level of care that is expected in a nursing home. Registration and inspection is undertaken by the local social services inspection unit.

73

There can be an overlap between the two types of care. There are bound to be some people who are in a residential home and need nursing care. It can be difficult to force somebody to move just at the moment when their health has deteriorated further. Some homes are able to deal with this problem by being dual-registered. That means that they have two adjoining sections, perhaps in neighbouring houses, with one offering basic care and the other nursing care, and transfers can be made without too much disturbance.

Homes specialising in dementia

During the 1990s there was a rapid increase in the number of homes specialising in dementia. One reason for this increase was the decline in the numbers of frail older people entering care. A change in registration from 'elderly' to 'elderly mentally ill' opens up the home to applications from a wider range of possible residents. As dementia becomes better known and the numbers of people with dementia increases, so the idea of accommodating this new group becomes more attractive. At the moment, however, it is not mandatory that the staff are trained afresh to meet the needs of this new client group.

Homes that are registered only for 'the elderly' nevertheless do often have people with dementia. The reason for this is partly that people develop dementia while they are living in a particular home and it would be unkind to make them move because they are now suffering from a new illness. It is also partly because there is no real requirement to keep to a particular category, even on admission.

> **Hazel** was living in a care home which was registered for people with a mental illness. As her physical condition got worse and she needed nursing care, she was transferred to a nursing home which was registered as an ordinary nursing home. A few months later she was followed by **Matilda** who had a similar health problem, needed greater physical care and had got to the stage where her dementia was so bad that she was unable to recognise people or places.

It can be hard for carers to find an appropriate home, especially as many are in a position where they need to find a place for a relative quickly. Finding out about staff training and attitudes towards people with dementia is vital in order to assess how this influences for good the way of life of the home – the way in which confused residents are spoken to, the way in which a disorientated older person is helped, the way in which family members are encouraged to understand what is going on in the mind of their relative.

Martin, the person in charge of a care home, talked at length to an agitated resident, **Rosemary**, about her fears that she was going to be removed from the home and sent somewhere else. This was not the home's plan and Martin was at pains to help Rosemary understand that there was no need to be afraid of a move which was not going to take place. He acknowledged the fear and tried to bring a measure of peace to a troubled older person.

Paying for long-stay care

Before somebody enters a care home, social services first make an assessment of needs. If it is decided that residential care is required, then they will make an assessment of means, according to national rules. As a result many people are responsible for paying their own fees, for example if they have investment income. Money from state benefits is also taken into account. In some cases the value of the house may be taken into account, but not if it is occupied by the spouse (or certain other people). Where there is capital below certain levels, the local authority is required to help towards paying the fees, according to national rules. If the family chooses a more expensive home, the difference will have to be paid by the resident or their spouse or family.

Some people may have their long-stay care fully funded by the NHS. This will be the case if they are 'sectioned' under certain sections of the Mental Health Act, and revised government guidance will set out health authority responsibilities for financing care. From October 2001, the nursing element of long-stay care will be fully funded by the NHS.

Social services are not required to pay for care at home if residential or nursing home care is a cheaper alternative that meets the person's needs. A 1995 High Court ruling allowed councils to limit their expenditure to take account of the available financial resources. It upheld the Lancashire

County Council decision to offer care in a nursing home rather than in the client's own home, indicating that there was no requirement for the local authority to pay out more money in order to satisfy the wishes of the individual or their family. However, from April 2002 the charging system is changing to try to minimise incentives for local authorities to use residential care and to tackle authorities which have a low cost ceiling in the amount of care they will provide at home.

Age Concern has a range of factsheets on residential care. For a list of factsheets contact the address on page 132.

Age Concern, the Alzheimer's Society and Counsel and Care all publish factsheets which give further details and up-to-date information about benefits and costs of care. Advice can also be obtained from Citizens' Advice Bureaux and from the Benefits Agency Helpline on 0800 882 200.

Costs of care

Economic analyses to date have been confined to the costs of Alzheimer's disease. Health service input is funded mainly from Community Mental Health Services budgets. Most public money is the responsibility of social services. A large percentage of the costs are carried by families and by social security, owing to the combination of benefits such as Attendance Allowance and the amounts that families pay through increased costs of care and the decreased opportunity to earn money themselves (see Chapter 6).

A 1997 study gave the following statistics:

- The average annual cost of care was £21,000, rising to £30,000 after nine years.
- A move to long-term care increased costs by £20,688 per year.
- The average opportunity cost (loss of earnings for example) was only £9,000 per year, with much higher costs where a person is diagnosed with dementia at an earlier age.
- The average cost of social services was £2,000–£2,500 per year.
- GP visits and outpatient appointments cost less than £100 a year.

(Economists Advisory Group 1997)

Pros and cons of long-stay care

There are advantages and disadvantages to both community care and long-stay care and much will depend on the ability of others to do the caring, and also on the amount of skill and memory that the individual has retained.

Matilda has considerable memory loss and is often confused. She does little cooking and cleaning, and needs to be helped with daily living activities.

Advantages of community care (ie care in own home, or in the home of a relative or a friend):

● Matilda will be surrounded by people and possessions that she may still recognise and value.
● She will not have the upheaval of a confusing move to a strange new environment.
● She will not be cut off from friends and neighbours.

Disadvantages of community care:

● Matilda is likely to require more help than can be provided by one carer all day (and night) all year round.
● She may lack stimulation as the carer is unlikely to have the energy to look after the house and help someone with dementia to be active as well.
● Community care may prove to be inadequate for her needs.
● There may be concerns for her safety in and out of the house.

Advantages of long-stay care:

● Matilda will be kept warm and dry; she will be fed and clothed. If the home is really good at looking after people (especially people with dementia) it will arrange suitable activities and outings.
● In many care homes, staff will be trained for the job.
● She will have company from other residents.
● She will be kept safer than in her own home.
● Her carer may be able to recover from the stresses of full-time caring.

Disadvantages of long-stay care:

- Matilda may be even more confused than usual by having to live in a strange place and with people she does not know. (This could be improved by previous attendance at a day centre in the same building.)
- Staff may have little idea of the needs of people with dementia.
- Finance may prove to be a problem both for Matilda and her family. It may be necessary to sell Matilda's house to cover her care costs.

Key points

■ Residential homes and nursing homes have different roles but there is considerable overlap between the two sectors.

■ Homes can register for 'elderly' or 'elderly mentally ill' residents but again in practice the two overlap.

■ Long-stay care can sometimes offer a more stimulating environment than the person's own home, provided that the care home understands the special needs of people with dementia.

Person-centred care

Negative attitudes to dementia care are disappearing and the concept of person-centred care has been key to this change. Good care improves standards by concentrating on the individual and not just on the illness. This section examines the characteristics of good care, including personalisation, privacy, choice and a reduction in the use of drugs. It highlights the need for *all* staff to be trained in dementia care problems and describes dementia care mapping, which can help give staff insight into the well-being of residents, and validation, which acknowledges feelings. The way in which a building is designed can also affect well-being and have a strong effect on the amount of risk that staff feel able to take. The section concludes by looking at the prevention of elder abuse.

Dementia care in the past

Negative attitudes to dementia care used to predominate, with the focus on the problems that dementia causes and the things that a person can no longer do:

> 'She was such a brilliant artist when she was younger. Now she has no idea what a brush is for.'

> 'He had a really good brain. He was an accountant in a big firm, but he had to retire early because of his illness. He couldn't manage to understand the job any longer.'

Comments like these are from carers who have seen a loved one disintegrate before their eyes; they naturally dwell on what has been lost, not on what has been retained and what can be brought back into action with enough stimulation and an appropriate environment.

The older styles of care were based on the belief that it is the person with dementia who is 'wrong'. People were labelled as 'wanderers', who were a problem and needed to be kept safely inside, or as 'aggressive' when they were confused and agitated by a world that they do not understand.

Care used to be found largely in the big geriatric and mental hospitals. The image was of a dead-end world with low-level nursing. Low staffing levels and low budgets gave poor self-esteem even where standards were high and there was excellent work being done. All too often the care lacked any imagination and people with dementia were kept in an environment where they were likely to be increasingly confused and increasingly made to be dependent on the staff who had a non-stop round of toileting, changing, washing and feeding. A low staff-to-patient ratio meant that it was necessary to use batch care methods; one nurse might have five or six people to feed at one time. Such a system might seem to be an efficient use of staff time, but it failed to understand the needs of people with dementia and treated them in a way that undermined any remaining self-esteem. The result was a loving care which led to more and more institutionalisation, dependency, aggression and change of personality. It was care on a medical model but without a medical answer.

Characteristics of the new culture of care

Personalisation

The old 30-bedded wards were no place for individual and personal possessions, but in modern care settings, residents can be surrounded by familiar objects:

> **Ravi** has a room with a view at his care home. The toilet is en suite, although he often expects it to be down the corridor. He has some of the furniture from his home, with a range of photos of family and friends. His favourite picture of the Lake District is near his bed. He feels at home, as he has been able to choose the decor himself. He is able to have his visitors there if he wants, although often he prefers to stay in the lounge or go into the garden. His front door is personalised. Ravi's name is written up, but there is a picture of a dog on the wall to remind him that this is his door. It also reminds him of the dogs he used to own.

Modern care enables people to be treated as individuals with the need to have connections with earlier parts of their lives, and to be treated with dignity and respect.

Personalisation involves:

- a private space to which others come by invitation; the staff do not have unrestricted right of access to a client's own area;
- encouraging the client and the family to bring the person's own furniture and other possessions, such as photos, souvenirs or a favourite cushion;
- 'way finders' for people to know that they have arrived at their own home: some indication at the door itself to show who lives there is helpful. (The staff may need to have the person's name, but the client may need to have a personalised, perhaps visual, indication to help choose the right door); and
- ideally the decor, or at least the pictures on the walls, should be chosen by the client.

Privacy

We all expect to have privacy in our lives, especially when it comes to washing, bathing and using the toilet. People with dementia have the same needs. They may appear to have lost their sense of modesty, but even those who have challenging behaviour will recognise the need for privacy at certain times. En-suite facilities in each room in care homes are a step towards recognising this need and giving much of the privacy and independence that everybody expects to have.

Choice

In the past people with dementia sometimes suffered what has been described as 'asset stripping'; ie they were subjected to a kindly regime in which the staff knew better than they did what they wanted. Thus there was no choice of food, for example; there was regimentation in the routines of life (such as the time to get up); and clothes were those provided by the hospital (and sometimes this meant nightclothes were kept on all day).

It is true that the complicated choices of many of our lives are not always possible for someone with dementia. For example, a choice of tea or coffee or hot chocolate, and 'by the way, you could have a cold drink as it is such a hot day', gives a muddled message that might confuse anybody. The key to success is a straight choice between two items: vegetables or salad; tea or coffee; ice-cream or trifle. There is the possibility that the person will answer by echoing the last item, but showing the two items may make it possible for the choice to be made by sight or by smell rather than just by words.

The same could apply to an activity – would you like to go for a walk in the park, or into town to look at the shops? Pictures of the park and the shops in town might enable the person to make a choice even though they may not understand the words that they are hearing.

Sexuality in dementia

A major issue for the care of people with dementia is the question of sexuality. Sexual behaviour does not come to an end with the onset of dementia. It may, however, become altered; indeed what previously may have been a delight and a joy, may become seen as a problem, or even as behaviour which is challenging. There may be an increased sexual drive on the part of the person with dementia, or, alternatively, there may be the opposite problem – a total lack of interest, or even a loss of interest or forgetfulness in the middle of sexual activity.

In a care home obvious expressions of sexual behaviour, such as masturbation, may cause distress or disgust to other residents and members of staff. Such behaviour needs to be treated with gentleness rather than seen as challenging, and certainly not stigmatised as 'dirty'. The person with dementia is unlikely to be aware of the feelings and attitudes of others, but may be missing out on intimacy. Some sexual behaviour is the result of a lack of inhibition, which is a characteristic of dementia, and needs to be understood as the result of disease even though it may be very frightening and upsetting to other residents.

Sexuality also includes opportunities for warmth and affection, caring and sharing. Often this can be absent in residential care, and two people may strike up a friendship which is at that level without causing eyebrows to be raised. Sharing a bed together may pose more of a problem, both morally and from the point of view of close family members. Care homes are not the guardians of anyone else's morals. As long as abuse is avoided, with consent on both sides, it is questionable whether care staff should intervene.

Reducing the use of drugs

The older forms of care tended to be linked to the regular use of drugs. When behaviour is seen as a problem which needs to be controlled, one method of coping is to administer tranquillising drugs.

There are homes which take people with the most challenging behaviours but use very few drugs. Homes which manage to cope without the use of drugs are characterised by many of the following features:

- The management philosophy is centred on the person and not on the illness.
- Staff training focuses on knowledge and understanding of dementia. There is an emphasis on standing in the shoes of the clients, trying to

feel what it might be like to be losing skills, faculties and memories, but also trying to get the person to make use of those memories and skills that remain.

- The training is not just for the care staff. It includes, for example, the cooks, the gardeners and the administrators. The managers receive ongoing training, as do the owners. (Training is looked at in more detail on pages 85–87.)
- The buildings are adapted for the needs of the person with dementia (see pages 87–90).
- Activities are suited to the needs of the individual who is encouraged to make an informed choice rather than just being told what to do (see Chapter 5). The same applies to choice of menu at mealtimes and the time of getting up and going to bed for example. Homes which are successful with 'difficult' clients are likely to be home in practice as well as in name.

For more information about person-centred care see Kitwood's book *The New Culture of Dementia Care* (1995).

Dementia care mapping

Inspectors of care homes do not have to evaluate the quality of the experience of residents with dementia. The aim of dementia care mapping (DCM) is to create a quality assurance scheme that measures the well-being of the client. It involves a team of two or three mappers whose job is to evaluate what the client experiences. It is done in five minute time-frames, with scores of:

- +5 (very good care)
- +3 (good care)
- +1 (maintenance care)
- −1 (slight ill-being)
- −3 (moderate ill-being)
- −5 (considerable ill-being)

Good care would indicate a positive interaction with someone else. A -3 incident might be a put-down by a member of staff involving a lack of respect for the person. A +5 incident is described as follows:

'Often this is where an interaction is evidently highly supportive of a person's self-worth, social confidence, personal control and hope.'
(Barnett 1995)

A member of staff takes her coffee break sitting with a very old woman who cannot speak but often utters repetitive little cries while looking round anxiously. Now they smile into each other's eyes, and the little cries become little laughs. Both persons seem to the observer to be enfolded in a warm and golden bubble of affection and happiness. After the caregiver has had to go back to work, the client continues to smile at the world, even reaching out a hand occasionally to touch those who pass by (Barnett 1995).

Part of the value of DCM is the focus on the quiet, the 'good' clients who cause no trouble, but who may be experiencing a state of ill-being which they deal with by becoming withdrawn and silent. The purpose of DCM is to enable staff to have an understanding of what is happening in a busy home, and to encourage them to adopt practices which lead to well-being. The mapping is something for which training is necessary, but which can be undertaken by anyone working in the home and also by home carers.

For further information about DCM and training courses, contact the Bradford Dementia Research Group at the address on page 123.

Validation

Good dementia care must acknowledge feelings. Validation means making valid, giving validity to, the feelings that people with dementia have. It means that we have to take seriously statements that we do not understand. It means that we must accept actions which seem to us to be bizarre. It means coming alongside someone and acknowledging the feelings behind the action or the words, even when we have to guess (and sometimes guess wrong).

Validation is the brainchild of an American woman called Naomi Feil. She talks about acknowledging and respecting the behaviour of very old disorientated people who express themselves poetically rather than logically (Feil 1982). Although, controversially, she believes that such people are not suffering from dementia, her approach to vulnerable people does encourage workers to operate on a 'feelings' level; discovering the feelings and acknowledging them can be a very effective way of helping the person to relax.

Many of the skills of validation are similar to those of good reflective counselling. The Feil method talks about training, and working at different levels of validation. It looks at universal symbols and what they can mean. For example, jewellery is a symbol of wealth and, not quite so obviously, a shoe might symbolise sex (along with many other items too). Actions take on new meaning – playing with faeces is not done to annoy the carer, but is viewed as a symbol of childhood pleasure.

The acknowledging of feelings is vital to the well-being of every person; dementia may even heighten that need. The whole person should be respected as of great value; the cultural traditions should be known, understood and respected; and a person's masculinity or femininity should also be prized. For example, a woman should be encouraged to wear clothes of the 'right' colour, and she should be able to have her hair done well and have her fingernails painted if she wishes.

Staff training and qualifications

Some of the nurses in nursing homes have a Mental Nursing qualification but most nurses do not have specific training in dementia. They may be very good at caring for people with severe physical illnesses but have no more knowledge of dementia than other care staff. Their training may even be a barrier to understanding the needs of people with dementia, as they may believe that there is nothing that medical skill can do for them and be completely unaware of the social aspects of care for which they will probably not have been trained at all.

Most care staff have few qualifications in dementia care as it is only relatively recently that there have been any qualifications towards which they could work. Further Education colleges and some specialist training establishments now offer courses in caring which attract large numbers of young women (if very few men) and lead to the NVQ qualification (National Vocational Qualification) and prepare students for careers in settings such as care homes. NVQ courses are also done in-house and are especially appropriate for older workers who were not offered any opportunity for initial training.

At the time of writing there is no module on dementia – a massive gap in provision which needs to be filled by those who devise such courses. There are, however, some dementia training courses on the market:

- The video-based course called *Care to Make a Difference* was designed by the Alzheimer's Society (address on page 121) for use within the workplace. There is an accreditation scheme with a certificate of achievement and a badge, both of which are awarded following a simple test. The value of this type of learning resource is that it can be undertaken by students on their own or in groups.
- *Dementia: A self-study pack* is produced by the Dementia Services Development Centre (DSDC) at Stirling University (address on page 128). Intended for individual study, it can also be used in group work and includes a video. No certification is offered.
- The DSDC in Stirling also runs regular one-day courses on a range of dementia issues. DSDCs are being established elsewhere in the UK, and some of them provide training courses – see the 'Useful addresses' section at the end of the book.

The most valuable training courses are often those which gather workers from different sectors of the care industry, as they enable a cross-fertilisation of experience and perception. In-house courses have the danger that the participants all know each other and can resist the messages which come across. There may also be distractions if someone has to go off in response to some sudden emergency.

Training is costly and if budgets have to be trimmed, training can be seen as something which is not really essential. In care homes and other care settings which cherish the new culture of dementia care, there is an accent on the training of *every* worker, as soon as they start work, including the gardener, the minibus driver, the cook, the young person who helps on a Saturday, and the volunteers. (Volunteers, of course, also need to be carefully vetted because of the vulnerability of people with dementia.) In these places the workers and their skills are valued and there is not so much chance for good work to be ruined by the inappropriate behaviour of even one member of staff.

In most jobs where people and their skills are valued, there is an accent on training before the new worker starts on the first day.

Building design

Around the world there are examples of buildings designed specifically for the needs of people with dementia.

As has already been mentioned on page 64, in parts of East Sussex there are day and respite centres refurbished specially for the needs of people with dementia. They are run by both social services and the health trust. Important features include:

- pleasant sitting areas decorated in pastel shades;
- walking routes inside the house which lead people back to where they started from;
- a house which feels more like a large private house or hotel than an institution;
- a garden which is safe to roam in; and
- a front door which is not locked during normal opening hours.

One of the houses in Sussex is set in a quiet street with not many obvious dangers for those who might go outside and get themselves lost. Another one has a walking route which enables residents to wander at will in a circle, even using the office as part of their route. People need opportunities to exercise and a walking route, inside or outside, helps people to get about without getting lost. Such a route cannot have frustrating dead-ends, but instead needs to be in the form of a loop or a series of loops so that the walkers always come safely back to the beginning.

Another of the Sussex homes has the disadvantage of being on a hillside with little garden space. However, the owners have catered for different client groups on the various floors. Each floor gives the impression of a pleasant and cheerful flat with good views out from the high ground. There is a kitchen available for residents to undertake some 'normal' activities under supervision and a small secure garden at the back.

None of these settings is absolutely ideal, but all have excellent features which make them into examples of good provision. What is essential is that people with dementia feel at home, and are made to feel useful. It is important to see dementia in terms of disability and to use this as the starting-point for all designs.

Problem	Design response
Poor (or no) memory	Compensate by building small units and creating circular routes.
Lack of confidence	Provide a domestic rather than an institutional setting. Use unobtrusive design features to help people know where they are.
Lack of individual identity	Incorporate cultural differences into design (for example a person's own furniture).
Inactivity	Enable residents to make use of the kitchen, help in the dining room, do craftwork, woodwork, gardening, look after animals, etc.

Some of the best design is to be found in the United States: Brawley, in her book *Designing for Alzheimer's Disease*, suggests the following:

- Design for units of eight people who are able to live together. Activities can then be seen from the person's door. A bigger scale makes it difficult for people with dementia to exercise choice.
- Colours need to be carefully chosen, so that a change in colour does not make it look as if there is a step, which leads to confusion.
- There should be no long corridors, especially not ending up with a fire escape.
- Corridors should always lead back to the starting point.
- If there are several corridors, each one should have a theme – for example, the seaside or animals – so that residents can identify their corridor easily.

(Brawley 1997)

Small rooms, where people can sit in twos and threes, create a feeling of cosiness. To alleviate hearing difficulties, curtains and other furnishings can be used to block out unwanted noises – planning the decor carefully is also important for people with eyesight problems. There also needs to be plenty of opportunities for residents to engage in their own activities (see Chapter 5). Thus there needs to be the space for such things as a washing line, an old car, or a garden shed for potting the plants.

If the building is to be a home for life, there needs to be some provision made for decline in a person's health and abilities. Residents who at first are able to energetically continue with their hobbies may eventually become unable to walk or even become bed-bound. Ideally they will continue to live in the same unit, and be looked after there until their death. This situation would be similar to people who were being looked after in the community in their own house. However, people who are admitted to care at a later stage of dementia may need to have a less domestic setting with space for items like hoists.

Locking the doors

'Wandering' can be a real problem for carers on their own, solved only by hiding the keys or putting bolts at the top of the doors or even (illegally) locking a loved one in the house so that the shopping can be done.

Although it should be different in long-stay care, in practice the emphasis is often on security, especially as it keeps carers and other members of the family happy and satisfies the home's duty of care.

During normal opening hours there should, however, ideally be no locked doors because:

- It is an abuse of a person's rights which do not vanish just because they have dementia. We do not lock people up just because they have a mental health problem, or because they do not conform to a particular way of life. We only do so within the framework of the Mental Health Act and the National Assistance Act. Neither of the Acts is designed for the needs of people with dementia who are living in care homes.
- Locking may make it easy to 'warehouse' residents, instead of offering them activities which are suited to their needs and the limitations that dementia has brought to their lives. 'Wandering' may be partly caused by boredom or merely the need to get out into the fresh air. Therefore, walkways should always be planned as part of the normal provision of any accommodation used by people with dementia.

- Locking increases the agitation of people who feel that they are being kept in against their will. It can cause the 'caged lion' effect and encourage people to be aggressive.
- Locking looks to the security of the person but avoids issues to do with the activities which are on offer.

Care homes do have a duty to care responsibly for residents. It is clearly irresponsible to allow out someone who is going to have an accident, but there is no need to eliminate all risks, as the law will only require that the person in charge has not been reckless or negligent in the execution of their responsibilities. Locking is more in line with the older culture of care which was designed for the benefit of the staff and the building rather than for the benefit of the clients.

There are alternatives to the lock and key approach which could be considered:

- A receptionist near the front door. Part of the job would be to keep an eye on the front door, and inform staff of anybody going out. Small homes might not be able to offer this; others would not have the space at the front door – it is questionable whether they are suitable establishments for the care of people with dementia.
- A warning device which is set off when someone opens the front door. There need be no loud bells; it can just be an alarm on a screen in the office.
- Using tagging devices which have the same effect as alarms. They are fitted to the person; but this should only be done with their permission.
- Encourage people to go out on their own, or with escorts in some cases, if they can be offered a circular route which they are still likely to be able to follow.

Preventing elder abuse

Abuse can take place in any setting – in residential care, in hospital, at the day centre, at the person's own home. Abuse happens to young people, to people with learning difficulties, to older people. Among older people, those with dementia are at great risk. It may be caused, not by a stranger, but by somebody who has some kind of relationship with an individual.

In a person's own home that is likely to be a member of the family. In a care home it may be a member of staff. Some abuse is intentional and planned; much is the result of frustration and the difficulty of dealing with a person whose behaviour has become too difficult to cope with. For all those who become involved with abuse, there is a need for understanding in two directions; firstly, an understanding of dementia and the behaviour that results from dementia, and, secondly, an understanding of the feelings that all carers have towards difficult people and difficult situations.

Abuse comes in different forms:

- physical
- psychological
- sexual
- financial

Dementia robs people of a real voice and also takes away their perception of what is happening. Carers (and others too) need to be ready to intervene but prevention is better than cure. The Alzheimer's Society has suggested measures that can be taken to enable both the family carer and the paid carer to cope with their roles, including:

- adequate support, including carers' support groups
- an environment suited to the needs of the person with dementia
- a culture of openness, where people are allowed to tell others what they are feeling
- monitoring of the health needs of family carers
- regular review by professionals of whether the carer can continue with the caring role
- assistance with dealing with difficult behaviour and situations
- advice on continence
- training on lifting and bathing
- adequate respite care

(Alzheimer's Society 1996)

Eastman suggests that the practice nurse should use the yearly check-up for people over the age of 75 as an opportunity to make use of the 'Cost of Care Index', which is a questionnaire focusing on the feelings that the carer is experiencing (Eastman 1994). A high score, indicating negative feelings, may show such a level of stress that professionals should intervene so as to prevent abuse happening.

In addition:

- paid staff need to be trained in dementia care, and given time to offload their concerns so that they can avoid the problems of burnout;
- purchasers of care (such as social services) need to monitor effectively;
- homes should be open to visits from friends and relatives at all reasonable times;
- the use of drugs and other forms of restraint should be open to independent scrutiny and not allowed to be a normal way of life; and
- financial abuse can be prevented in homes by ensuring that there is independent checking of accounts.

Above all, abuse can be avoided by expecting staff and family carers to seek the consent of the person with dementia for decisions in their lives, including advance consent for the time when they are no longer able to communicate their wishes. Action on Elder Abuse (address on page 121) operates a confidential helpline service providing information for anyone and emotional support for those involved.

Key points

■ Good dementia care is centred on the person and not on the illness.

■ Its characteristics are: personalisation; privacy; choice; and having a range of activities available.

■ Good care reduces the need for drugs.

■ All staff need to be trained in dementia care principles.

■ Dementia care mapping enables staff to focus on the well-being or ill-being of individual clients.

■ Validation is a skill which helps in the acknowledgement of feelings.

- Not all staff in care homes are qualified and trained, but increasing numbers now have a National Vocational Qualification (NVQ). There is no NVQ dementia module, but courses on dementia are available.

- Buildings should be designed for the needs of people with dementia.

- All frail people are at risk from abuse. It can be prevented in most settings through adequate staff training and support.

CHAPTER 5

Activities for people with dementia

Like everyone else, people with dementia need to be kept stimulated. This chapter suggests that a range of activities will offer opportunities for them to exercise choice and to fulfil their potential. Reality Orientation or reminiscence can be helpful, as can sensory stimulation or the use of music. The chapter concludes with a consideration of spiritual needs.

A range of activities

Having choice in the activities that are available gives opportunities to people with dementia to make use of the skills that they still have. Art and music classes may result in even the most withdrawn of people beginning to show an interest and take part in their own way.

Similarly, it should be possible to involve people with dementia in some of the activities of the kitchen and the dining room. They could for example be offered the chance of setting the table or clearing up after a meal. There may be opportunities for doing some gardening, woodworking or tinkering around with an old car. Normalisation policies in care homes enable people to undertake simple domestic tasks without it being seen as a threat to either the routine of a home or a problem with regard to health and safety.

A good day centre or care home provides a range of activities that people can choose from, suitable for men as well as women. Some people prefer to play a game of patience on their own, while others may be happy to join in a ball game activity or a bingo session. Other ideas, for experiences which are good for the spirit, mind and body, include:

- a coach trip to see the Christmas lights
- a concert in the village hall
- visits from the local school choir
- joint painting sessions with local children
- a chance to visit the countryside or look at the stars

Groups can be booked on a professional basis. The North Tyneside branch of the Alzheimer's Society received funding to employ a professional artist to encourage the creation of a mural. This project involved both people with dementia and carers. Themes were chosen to represent aspects of dementia; for example, a magpie with a ring in its beak represents the hoarding tendency of many people with dementia. It was not necessary for people to have great artistic ability, as some were able just to do basic leaves and flowers (Neal 1996).

Group exercise sessions help to maintain physical fitness, and there are trained and qualified exercise professionals available to undertake such activities, including chair-based activities. The teacher should be on the professional Exercise register of England (with similar bodies in Wales, Scotland and Northern Ireland). A company in Leeds called JABADAO uses dance to create a movement language which can be the only expression of feelings and needs for some residents, bringing with it a confidence that may be lacking with words and a release from tensions.

Reality Orientation

Reality Orientation (RO) is one activity which aims to bring understanding to people who have difficulty remembering the basic information of life. At its most simple it is a technique which can help people to be reminded of the following:

- other people's names
- where they are living now

- the time of day
- the day of the week
- the month of the year
- the weather now
- what the next meal is going to be

Some of that information can be provided as part of ordinary conversation. It can also be done as an RO session. This is sometimes the job of an Occupational Therapist (OT). It may take half an hour or so for an OT to go through the programme with half a dozen people. Some homes and day centres use an RO board to help as a memory jogger; in this case, however, people must be able to read and understand what they read, and the information must be up-to-date.

Other workers use a more extensive version of RO to jog people's memories about facts that they may have difficulty in remembering. For example, they may not be able to recall the names of the flowers that are blooming in the garden. Good RO technique would be to introduce this into the conversation ('Those tulips look lovely today'). Alternatively, a formal session might cover a topic such as money or shopping.

RO attempts to deal with a cognitive deficit. The information will inevitably be forgotten in hours, if not in minutes. On its own it does not meet people's underlying needs. Nonetheless it is valuable as a tool for workers, especially when it is used in regular conversation, or as a way of greeting a person in the morning and of reminding them where they are and who you are.

Speechmark Publishing is one company which produces materials to support RO activities – the address is on page 125.

Reminiscence

It used to be thought harmful to remind people of things from the past. It may be that life's events have been so hard for some people that they are distressed by thinking back for example to family members whom they have lost. For most people, however, a careful selection of photos of people and places from the past brings pleasure and lifts the spirits. It helps to unlock memories and gives an opportunity for conversation. It makes older people feel experts again.

Photos belonging to the person with dementia are the most helpful. They tell of their own family, workplace, or village where they were brought up. They evoke memories of special days and places, memories which are highly valuable for those who have few memories left.

Local postcards and photos from old newspapers are of particular value for people who have lived in the same town all their life. For those who started life in another part of the country it is always possible to get similar photos after a search through *Yellow Pages* to find the right sort of dealer in old pictures. There are also commercially produced photos – for example Speechmark Publishing produces a range of material including a 'Then and Now' series. This series shows pictures of old and modern versions of the same thing; for example a bus in 1920 and a bus today, or a telephone from the turn of the century and a modern one. Age Exchange (address on page 121) sells large photographs of events from the past, for example people going on an outing in a charabanc or pictures of shops and schools. Age Exchange also offers courses and holds conferences on reminiscence.

For further information see the Age Concern Books publications *Reminiscence and Recall: A guide to good practice* and *The Reminiscence Trainer's Pack*. Further details are given on pages 130–131.

Sensory stimulation

A special room set aside for the purpose of relaxation and stimulation is the basis for work with people with dementia who may have difficulty with other forms of communication. The idea comes from work done with people with learning difficulties in the Netherlands where the Dutch word *snoezelen* (sniff and doze) is used. The sensory experiences include:

- lighting effects
- soft music
- aromatherapy
- massage
- touching of various sorts of textures

The results are sometimes dramatic in reducing agitation and challenging behaviour. It is also an activity which can involve the staff.

A study of work done at King's Park Community Hospital in Bournemouth showed the beneficial and calming effect on 12 patients (Benson 1994). All 12 were suffering from severe ·dementia and were exhibiting behaviour problems which could not be managed in nursing homes. The 'sniff and doze' sessions were not only helpful to the patients, but also popular with the staff.

Music

Many people with dementia retain their music memory for a much longer period of time than their language memory. Indeed it can be the music that unlocks the memory and triggers off all the words of a popular song or well-known hymn. The result can be amazement that someone who is regarded as having no speech can suddenly remember all the words. Music can also have a soothing and calming effect on people with dementia. It must, however, be the music of their choice, or at least music which the carer believes is their choice.

Local choirs can be invited to day centres and care homes. Concerts can be particularly successful if the choir chooses a programme appropriate to the needs of the audience, and offers an opportunity for people to join in with old favourites as well as performing their usual repertoire. Those who have an instrumental skill should be encouraged to continue with it (or take it up again). It is good for the fine movements of the hand, and may be good entertainment for others too.

Dance can also be a powerful means of unlocking the memory. There have been occasions when people in wheelchairs have suddenly got to their feet and started dancing, spurred on by the music they are hearing. Dancing also gives the opportunity for human contact and physical activity.

Spiritual needs

Some people will want an opportunity for worship similar to their experiences in previous years. Long-stay hospitals used to have a chapel and chaplain; closure and transfer to care homes has removed this element of the spiritual and often there has been nothing to replace it. So for many people in care homes there is nothing to remind them of worship and faith unless they continue to be visited by members of their church. Such a visit still does not give the chance of worship together with others, unless a visit to church can be arranged. It might be better if it could be organised within the home itself.

> **Madge** says loudly that she wants a sweet. Care worker Gary shares a large-print hymn sheet with her. He points to each word with his finger, and she sings some words. She appears to be concentrating hard, and forgets about the sweet for a few minutes. **Josef** and **Frank** listen in, half asleep. It is difficult to tell what value the service is to them, but Gary is reminded of the woman a year ago who also seemed to be asleep and then said how wonderful the singing had been. Gary felt that it had created a heavenly quality for her. **Jacob** comes by; he seems to have no idea what is happening. **Alicia** has taken a copy of the hymn sheet and is making her way through it. She talks a language of her own that Gary does not understand, but she has been present and it is not for him to say it has been a waste of time.

If running such a service:

- Keep it short. One or two points referring to something familiar will be enough.
- Use visual aids (such as candles at Christmas). Give people something to hold and talk about (perhaps harvest items at the end of the summer). Bring objects that have a nice smell (perhaps perfume or fruit to illustrate a story).
- Use mainly old, well-known hymns.
- Read a short passage from the Bible, preferably something well-known, such as a parable or a popular psalm.
- Try to get residents to take part, perhaps through things that they remember from the past. For example, they may be able to tell you something about their own faith.

These points relate to a Christian service but the same principles will apply to people from other world faiths. They will also respond to those things that are familiar and to words and rituals that have been part of their life both as children and adults.

It is important that people with dementia can also make a choice whether they want to be in the main room during the service or not. If they want to walk out after five minutes, that should be acceptable to those who have come to take the service. On the other hand nobody should be left out, unless that is their choice.

Key points

■ Having choice in the activities that are available will give opportunities to people with dementia to make use of the skills that they still have.

■ Activities for people with dementia include: exercise; Reality Orientation; reminiscence; and sensory stimulation.

■ Music may be a good way of bringing a soothing atmosphere, and may also unlock the speech memory.

■ There should be opportunities for worship suited to the needs of people with dementia.

Home carers

This chapter highlights some of the challenges involved in caring for someone with dementia. It looks at the isolation that carers can experience, role reversal, back problems and financial difficulties. Faced with these problems, it is not surprising that some people become frustrated, angry and distressed, and these difficult feelings are often themselves a source of guilt. However, with experience, information and support, many problems can be avoided or solved, or their impact reduced. The chapter concludes by highlighting the positive aspects of caring for someone.

Isolation

Although health and social services have a vital role to play in the care of people with dementia, for those living at home most of the necessary day-to-day practical and emotional support is provided by their family and friends. There are many reasons why people become carers: some slip into the role almost without noticing as the dementia progresses; for some it may be unavoidable; for a few there may be a financial motive. For most people, however, caring is a willing duty of love that they expect and want to do. An important function of formal health and social care is to enable carers to continue in this role for as long as they are able and willing to do so. Providing this support can sometimes be difficult; even when the tasks become burdensome, many carers are reluctant to give up the intimate care of their loved one to strangers. However, the best care usually results from families and services working together in partnership.

Looking after someone with dementia can be very demanding – physically, emotionally and financially. It can also be very lonely. Community care gives the impression of neighbours and friends rallying round to support the family in its hour of need. The phone rings regularly to ask how the person is getting on. People offer lifts in their car, children are picked up from school by other parents, someone bakes a cake for a family under pressure. Although this may be true in a crisis, all too often carers know little of this kind of support six months after their caring role starts. A form of compassion fatigue can set in when it appears that the 'emergency' is going to be permanent.

> When his wife **Rose** was admitted for assessment, **Godfrey** was taken to the hospital every day by a number of friends. Three years later he was still visiting every day, but now he was spending an hour or so, and travelling partly on foot and partly with two buses. Friends were still around for emergencies, but now it was just as much part of Godfrey's everyday life as it was when he caught the bus to work in the morning.

Dementia is still a taboo subject for many people and carers sometimes find that friends and even family members stop calling. The carer is less and less able to get out and about – a quiet drink in the pub is out of the question; even going to the shops is a matter of a quick dash and no time to talk.

Going out with the person they are caring for can present even more problems.

> The mini-market had the usual sweets and other attractive items on display by the checkout. **Maurice** slipped a chocolate bar into his pocket while his daughter **Georgia** was not looking. But one of the staff saw the manoeuvre and challenged the shoplifter. Maurice was completely confused by the chaos. Georgia was embarrassed that her dad should have tried to steal.

Going out can present a range of unexpected hazards to the carer. It can be easier in a small town or village or in a local shopping parade. There the carer needs to pluck up the courage to tell the shop owner and staff that their relative is suffering from dementia and sometimes behaves in unexpected ways. It is unlikely then that the shop will call for the police and insist on a prosecution. Bigger shops are less easy to deal with and constant vigilance may be required to avoid embarrassing incidents.

Using public transport may also present difficulties:

> **Troy** thought it would be a good idea to go into town on the new minibus that served his village. What he had not bargained for was his mother **Beryl**'s refusal to get on board to come home again. In the end Troy resorted to pushing her on and taking no notice of the fuss she was making (and the look on the faces of the other passengers).

There is also the problem of using public toilets:

> For **Mavis** it was a nightmare every time her husband **Albert** needed to 'go'. She could hardly go with him into the men's loo near the station. So she waited and hoped that he would manage on his own. One day she waited 20 minutes before she finally had to ask a male passer-by to help. Albert had completely forgotten that his wife was waiting outside for him. He thought he had to wait for her to come for him. That was no big problem for the passer-by, but he might have had a dressing or even cleaning up job to do, which might have been seen as beyond the call of duty.

Such problems may discourage carers so much that they may stay at home as much as possible and avoid taking the risks that lead to an embarrassing or difficult situation in public. RADAR runs a national toilet key scheme, further details of which can be obtained by phoning 020 7250 3222.

Many carers value their carers' support group. The group may be part of the Alzheimer's Society (address on page 121) or Carers National Association (address on page 123), or it may be run by a day centre or a care home. Support groups give members an opportunity to talk about their situation and learn from each other, and perhaps also have outings or help to arrange social occasions. However, there is still a need for neighbours and friends to keep aware of carers and not drop them in favour of people who are more able to get out and about.

Bereavement

'Out of sight, out of mind' becomes a feature of any carer's life unless they are surrounded by a large and loving family, or else have a supportive network of friends. For people looking after someone with dementia there may be the additional experience of losing a companion:

'It's like living with a stranger'

'There's no conversation any longer'

'I'm really on my own here in the flat'

We normally think of bereavement as something linked with the death of a person. With people who have dementia, the body may stay alive for many years after they themselves seem to have departed from it. There may be times when the 'old' person is back again, but that usually only lasts a brief moment before vanishing again.

Carers say things like:

'My husband died two years ago. But his body is still living and I have to carry on looking after its needs.'

'I shed my tears on the way back home from visiting Dad. So, when he died there weren't any more tears left.'

It is difficult to deal with any terminal illness. With many conditions it may be possible to communicate, make plans and get affairs in order. With dementia, communication may be something that only happens rarely; indeed there may seem to be no response or awareness. While some carers manage to keep on visiting to the end, others become discouraged and upset, and stay away.

Role reversal

The children of people with dementia may find themselves having to take care of their parent. It is often men and women in middle life who are faced with an elderly parent who no longer has the capacity to cope with ordinary life. The most intimate of activities, like toileting and washing, may thus need to be undertaken by the carer. It is a reversal of the normal role when a son has to take his mother to the toilet and clean her bottom. 'I'd never seen my mother with no clothes on' is what one middle-aged man said about the situation in which he found himself. It is no different for a daughter, who is more likely to take on the carer role than her brother anyway. It is just as difficult to have to persuade Mum or Dad to get undressed and have a bath. It is the reverse of the normal relationship between a parent and a child, even when the child has become an adult, and it can put the carer's mental health at risk. It can also put strains on the carer's marriage and other relationships.

Younger children as carers

Younger children of people with dementia may have their teenage lives upset by a parent or grandparent who behaves in a bizarre manner. They may decide that it is not possible to invite friends home to the house, especially if there is any chance that Dad is going to make a scene. Or they may find themselves in situations which are beyond their coping ability.

Jade was 16 when she agreed to mother-sit for an hour while her father went out for a quick drink. All of a sudden Mum decided that she was going for a walk – despite the rain outside. Before Jade knew what was happening, she was at the front door trying to stop her Mum from leaving. There was a huge row, with Mum wanting to know who she thought she was telling her own mother to stay in the house. They were both in tears, when the next-door neighbour heard the commotion and came to give a hand.

It might have been better if Jade had been more patient. She could perhaps have tried to persuade her mother not to go, instead of arguing, or else she could have gone for a walk round the block despite the rain. She was taken by surprise, however, and tried to exercise her authority as the person in charge. It was a long time before Jade felt able to look after her mother again on her own. If young people are involved in caring, it is important to involve them in decision-making and to take their views into consideration.

Back problems

Carers also have to deal with a range of practical issues. The later stages of dementia can introduce new problems for carers. Instead of being up and about at all hours of the day and night, the person with dementia may become unable to move by themselves. This may be as a result of a fall, some other condition such as arthritis, or by the person forgetting how to walk or how to sit down in a chair.

The result can be a heavy load for carers who may themselves be getting frail. To lift an adult on your own is contrary to health and safety regulations. Yet these regulations only apply to people who are employed. Thus

carers regularly do a lifting job that younger care workers are not permitted to do. In addition they do it without the benefit of training and often
without the benefit of equipment which could take a weight off their
backs. Not surprisingly, some carers suffer from back problems; some
have to stop caring altogether because they are no longer capable of doing
the necessary lifting.

Finances

For many home carers financial problems are a great worry. Carers
ususally receive no pay; indeed, when they go on holiday they may have
to pay someone else to do their job. That can apply to respite care in day
centres or residential homes and also (if you can find them) to people
who will come into your home and live on the job.

There may be unexpected extra expense when there is someone in the
family to be looked after:

- there can be more damage and wear and tear than usual;
- incontinence may result in clothing or carpets having to be replaced;
- accidents can happen to property;
- things of value may be thrown away, even banknotes burned on the
  fire; and
- transport costs may increase.

Caring costs the carer money anyway. Some people give up a job to care,
or only work part-time, resulting in a lower income and probably a lower
pension at retirement age. Invalid Care Allowance (see below) may be a
help but it does not make up for a regular wage or salary.

How much a person is expected to pay for social services usually depends
on the amount of capital that they have. Anyone with a house can expect
to have to fund residential and nursing home care through the sale of the
property unless their spouse or a dependant is living there (see pages
75–76).

Whether or not it is cheaper to care for someone at home depends on the
level of service that is needed. Round-the-clock care can be very expensive and local authorities are not bound to provide it just because

someone expresses the wish to stay in their own home. Social services are responsible for assessing the need of a person and also their ability to pay. Although there are national rules for charging for residential and nursing home care, each local authority is able to decide whether and how much to charge for care at home.

> For more information see Age Concern Factsheet 41 *Local Authority Assessments for Community Care Services.* For more information about paying for residential or nursing home care, Age Concern has a range of factsheets. For a list of factsheets contact the address on page 132.

Day centres and respite care may also need to be paid for. Transport costs may be high, particularly if taxis have to be hired for any outing. Attendance Allowance (see below) may help to pay for some things, but otherwise the breaks have to be paid for by the person with dementia and their family. This may discourage people from using services, and reduce their viability.

Social security benefits

Many people have no idea of the world of benefits before illness strikes. First of all it is the responsibility of care professionals to make sure that the carer is pointed in the right direction. However, the GP is not likely to be an expert on benefits. An alternative is for people to contact the social services department, which is responsible for assessing the client (the person with dementia) and also the carer. You can always go direct to the Benefits Agency, but you are only likely to do that if you know what to ask for in the first place. The best option may be to get in contact with one of the agencies which specialise in benefits advice, such as a Citizen's Advice Bureau, or an appropriate voluntary organisation locally such as Age Concern.

Disability Living Allowance (DLA) has a mobility component and an attendance component. To qualify people have to become ill or disabled and make a claim before the age of 65. You claim **Attendance Allowance** if you are 65 or over. The amount that is granted depends on the level of care that has to be given (there are day and night-time conditions).

These benefits are paid to the person with the disability, whereas **Invalid Care Allowance** is paid to carers. From 2001 it is available to all carers but there is a limit to the amount that the carer is able to earn. The carer is eligible for Invalid Care Allowance only if the person they are looking after is receiving Attendance Allowance or DLA.

Carers living on a low income may also be entitled to Income Support and Housing Benefit, which are both means-tested benefits and can include an extra 'carer premium' amount.

For more information about benefits, see Age Concern Factsheet 18 *A Brief Guide to Money Benefits* or Factsheet 34 *Attendance Allowance and Disability Living Allowance*, or contact the Benefits Helpline on Freephone 0800 88 22 00.

Council Tax

People may be exempt from paying Council Tax if:

- they have a doctor's certificate saying that they have a 'severe mental impairment'. They also have to be receiving a benefit such as Attendance Allowance; or
- they are looking after someone with an illness such as dementia for at least 35 hours a week. The person, however, must not be a husband, wife, partner or a child less than 18 years old. The person being cared for must be receiving a benefit such as Attendance Allowance at the highest rate.

Further information and advice can be obtained from the Council Tax department of the local authority or see Age Concern Factsheet 21 *The Council Tax and Older People*.

Enduring Power of Attorney

People with dementia may eventually become unable to cope with financial matters. As soon as it is clear that someone is suffering from dementia, the carer should organise an Enduring Power of Attorney. Power of attorney is a device which gives one person the right to look after another person's financial affairs for them. The person giving the power must be of sound mind and be able to understand the effect of signing the document, which should still be possible at an early stage of dementia.

Information and application forms can be obtained direct from the Public Trust Office (address on page 125). Employing a solicitor might be a good idea, especially one who understands the problems of dementia, such as the ones working within the Alzheimer's Society's LAWNET scheme. Contact the national office of the Alzheimer's Society for a list of those taking part in the scheme (England, Wales and Northern Ireland only) – see address on page 121.

The powers of an attorney are restricted to financial matters. It is a good idea to consult other family members at an early stage, so that they are kept in the picture throughout. In any case relatives are able to make objections before the Enduring Power of Attorney is registered, and they can also make their complaints to the Public Trust Office at a later stage if they believe that the donor's affairs are not being looked after properly.

The Court of Protection

Some carers realise too late that they should have arranged for an Enduring Power of Attorney to be signed. Their relative or friend may suddenly have become incapable of signing the form, or understanding what they are doing. The bank may realise the situation and refuse to honour cheques.

The way forward is to apply to the Court of Protection to appoint the carer (or a friend or relative) as 'receiver' (someone who is made responsible for the financial affairs of someone who is no longer mentally capable). The Court will need to make enquiries about the medical condition of the person with dementia and also details about the family. Receivers are required to act in the best interests of the person they are acting on behalf of. They are accountable to the Court of Protection, which charges a fee for its services.

Clearly it is best to avoid the need to apply to the Court of Protection as its enquiries take time; the Enduring Power of Attorney saves a lot of worry and is less expensive.

Where a person with dementia is entitled to social security benefits or allowances, a person (usually a close relative) may be appointed to make claims for and receive benefits on their behalf.

The Alzheimer's Society has an information sheet entitled *Financial and Legal Arrangements* and Age Concern Factsheet 22 is called *Legal Arrangements for Managing Financial Affairs*.

A positive experience

Caring can be a source of great satisfaction. It may bring the family together to agree on how they are going to share out the responsibilities. Indeed it may give the opportunity for young and old to work together and not just concern themselves with their own interests. For children it may be an experience which forms character and personality – there may be a special bond forged between a grandparent and grandchild; it may result in opening up career opportunities in the caring professions; or it may just make a teenager more aware of the needs of others around them.

It is important for the whole family, children included, to be aware of what happens to the brain of someone with dementia. Reading a book like the Alzheimer's Society's guide for families and other carers *Caring for the Person with Dementia* (Woods and Lay 1996) may be a great help. *It's Me, Grandma, it's Me* (Evans 1991) is a book for primary school children. Such publications can help to give knowledge and understanding which empowers carers of all ages, and ensure that they are able to ask professionals useful and even challenging questions.

Key points

- Family carers experience a range of normal emotions such as anger.
- They also experience unusual feelings as a result of a reversal of roles and a sense of bereavement while their relative is still alive.
- Family problems can arise when a person with dementia is added to the household.
- Caring for someone is expensive.
- Carers may be eligible for the social security benefit Invalid Care Allowance and/or exemption from Council Tax.

- An Enduring Power of Attorney will enable the financial affairs of the person with dementia to be looked after when they are no longer able to understand them.
- Caring is a positive experience for many people.

CHAPTER 7

Into the future

The final chapter looks ahead at what the future holds in terms of service development and scientific advances. The book concludes with some aims for the future.

Around the world

Over the last two decades there have been great improvements in the field of dementia care, but there is still much to do. In the developed world, the number of people with dementia will continue to increase for many years to come, and services will need to expand and develop to keep up. Other social trends, such as the increasing numbers of people who live alone, will also create new challenges that services will have to meet.

In the developing world, the challenge is considerably greater. Many countries with traditionally small older populations are now experiencing rapid ageing, and a corresponding increase in the numbers of people with dementia. Health services often have no resources to manage this new problem, particularly where services and policies are geared to reducing infant mortality. Popular awareness and understanding of dementia is low, and support groups are few, although groups such as Alzheimer's Disease International are working hard to encourage their development. In these countries it will be the families and local communities who will have to carry the burden of care for the foreseeable future.

Service development in the UK

The UK has specialist old age psychiatry services in most districts, but the provision of dementia care in primary health care and social care is still very uneven, and this will have to improve if the needs of people with dementia and their carers are to be met. In general, all services are still too inflexible, poorly co-ordinated and insufficiently sensitive to the wishes and opinions of those they serve.

A number of national policy developments currently under way in the UK have the potential to deliver significant change in the way that dementia services are organised and experienced by patients and carers. In particular, the move towards a primary-care-led NHS and the development of Primary Care Groups (PCGs) and Primary Care Trusts (PCTs) will result in a very different mechanism for the commissioning and delivery of services. In future, it will be the PCTs which draw up the service plans for dementia care.

Another major impetus for change will be the National Service Framework for Older People, which will set out, in broad terms, how services should be organised and delivered. There is an increasing emphasis on the quality and effectiveness of services, with groups such as the Commission for Health Improvement, the Social Care Institute of Excellence (SCIE) and the National Institute of Clinical Excellence (NICE) being set up to pronounce on these. It remains to be seen just how effective they will be in improving standards in dementia care.

Scientific advances

Even less predictable is what the future will bring in terms of scientific and technological solutions to the problem of dementia. The pace of research is now extremely fast, and has the potential to deliver some fundamental treatments, although these are probably some decades away. Possible treatment strategies in the future include: drugs to prevent the build-up of the toxic proteins, such as beta-amyloid, that kill nerve cells in Alzheimer's disease; a vaccine against beta-amyloid; and even replacement of lost nerve cells by implants. However, they will all require extensive testing to see if they are effective, safe and acceptable to patients.

The ultimate goal is to treat dementia before it becomes clinically apparent, or to prevent it occurring in the first place. Pre-clinical treatment will require not only an effective intervention (see above), but also a means of screening for the disease, and there are as yet no simple blood tests for conditions such as Alzheimer's. A better understanding of the factors that increase and decrease the risk of developing dementia may lead to effective prevention strategies. For example, there is evidence to suggest that anti-inflammatory drugs and oestrogens may reduce the risk of developing Alzheimer's disease. However, these hypotheses need to be rigorously tested in long-term studies before they can be recommended for clinical use. It is also possible that dietary interventions such as vitamin B12 and folic acid supplements, lowering cholesterol levels, daily aspirin, or even moderate wine consumption, may be of value (Smith 1998), but here also much more research is needed. Many of the risk factors for vascular dementia (smoking, high blood pressure, diabetes) are already well-known. These patients are also likely to benefit from regular low-dose aspirin, which thins the blood and reduces the risk of future mini-strokes.

New treatments for dementia will have important consequences for service provision. Even now, health services are having to change in order to accommodate the first generation of anti-Alzheimer drugs. Increased demand and earlier presentation of the illness will require improved diagnostic skills, and patients and carers will need to have easy and equitable access to appropriate treatment and care. The immediate challenge is to find the right balance, in terms of both effectiveness and cost, between the new health technologies and high quality community and long-term residential care. In achieving this, it is crucial that the voice of the carer and the patient are heard.

Aims for the future

Alzheimer Europe has produced a document called 'Declaration of needs and rights for people with dementia and their carers'. Key aims include:

- People with Alzheimer's disease need accurate and timely diagnosis.
- Carers and family members need recognition of their special role in the provision of care.

- People with dementia need a range of health and social care provision, such as respite for caregivers and sensitive and appropriate care for the dying.
- The social security and welfare systems of each country should ensure financial support for younger people with dementia and their families.
- Public awareness and education is the basis of improved care for people with dementia through education and training.
- Research is essential to improve care, develop therapies and ultimately find a treatment and cure. It should involve people with dementia and their families as active participants.

(Alzheimer Europe 1998)

The following aims could also be added, based on the information in this book:

- All doctors should update their understanding and awareness of dementia, so that patients are not prevented from obtaining diagnosis and support.
- Families should be offered a range of support services (sitters, day care, respite care) with costs falling more on the community and less on the family.
- Care homes should provide accommodation and activities designed for person-centred care.
- All staff dealing with people with dementia should have dementia training before they start their work, as well as in-service training. This training should apply to care staff who visit people in their own homes, and also to all staff and volunteers in care homes and day centres.
- The needs of younger people with dementia should be specially catered for.
- Information about dementia should be readily available in high streets and supermarkets, and also in surgeries.
- The voice of people with dementia should increasingly be heard.

Key points

■ In the developing world, health services are not well-placed to cope with increasing numbers of people with dementia.

■ The provision of dementia care in the UK needs to be more flexible and responsive and better co-ordinated.

■ A number of national policy developments will help bring about change in the organisation of dementia services in the UK.

■ Fundamental treatments and prevention strategies are probably still decades away but more drug treatments are likely to become available.

■ New treatments for dementia will have important consequences for service provision.

■ It is important that the voice of people with dementia be heard.

Glossary

Admiral Nurses Specialists in dementia care, operating an 'at home' service in certain areas.

Alzheimer's disease Main form of dementia.

Amyloid Poisonous protein in the brain.

Arteriosclerosis Disease caused by hardening of the arteries.

BSE A spongiform dementia (where the brain takes on a sponge-like texture) in cattle.

Community Psychiatric Nurse (CPN) Specialist in mental illness.

Creuzfeldt-Jakob Disease (CJD) A rare spongiform dementia. In its new variant form it has been described as the human version of 'mad cow disease'.

Crossroads A care attendant scheme, available in many areas of the UK, offering a home care service.

Dementia care mapping System of quality control used in some establishments looking after people with dementia.

Down's Syndrome A condition which causes learning difficulties. People with Down's Syndrome have an increased risk of getting Alzheimer's disease.

Early-onset dementia Describes dementia in people under the age of 65.

EMI (elderly mentally infirm) Used to describe a care home which takes older people with mental health problems, including dementia.

Hippocampus Small part of the back of the brain which is involved in memory storage.

Huntington's Chorea A genetic dementia.

Korsakoff's Syndrome Rare dementia linked to alcoholism.

Late-onset dementia Dementia in people aged 65 and over.

Lesion Damage to brain tissue.

Lewy-Body Disease Dementia which has some features similar to Parkinson's Disease.

Multi-infarct dementia Dementia resulting from many small strokes.

Neuro-fibrillary tangles Twisted molecules made of protein found within the nerve cells. They cause degeneration of neurones.

Neurone Brain cells involved in the transmission of nerve impulses.

NVQ (National Vocational Qualification) A qualification which some care assistants have or are working towards.

Pick's Disease A dementia of the frontal lobes of the brain.

Plaque Unusual feature in the brain connected with poisonous protein.

Pre-senile Out-of-date term for early-onset dementia.

Prions Infectious proteins involved in the development of CJD.

Pseudo-dementia A condition which has similar features to dementia, but which can be controlled and in some cases cured.

Reality Orientation A system for encouraging people with dementia to retain their information skills.

Respite care Holiday care service which enables the carer to have a break.

Senile Out-of-date term for an old person with dementia.

Snoezelen Dutch word used to describe sensory experiences used in some settings for people with dementia.

Validation Care concept which highlights empathy in dealing with people with dementia.

Vascular disease Damage to the blood vessels. If the oxygen supply fails in the brain, brain cells may die, possibly leading to strokes or multi-infarct dementia.

Bibliography

Alzheimer Europe (1998) 'Declaration of needs and rights of people with dementia and their carers'. *Alzheimer Europe Newsletter*, 1 December 1998.

Alzheimer's Society (1996) *Mistreatment of People with Dementia and their Carers*. Alzheimer's Society: London.

Barnett E (1995) 'A window of insight into quality care'. *Journal of Dementia Care*, July 1995.

Bell J and McGregor I (1995) 'A challenge to stage theories of dementia'. In: Kitwood and Benson (eds) *The New Culture of Dementia Care*. Hawker: London.

Benson S (1994) 'Sniff and doze therapy'. *Journal of Dementia Care*, January 1994.

Bosanquet N et al (1998) *Alzheimer's Disease in the United Kingdom: Burden of disease and future care*. Health Policy Unit, Imperial College School of Medicine: London.

Brawley E (1997) *Designing for Alzheimer's Disease*. John Wiley: Bognor Regis.

Burns A et al (1995) *Alzheimer's Disease: A medical companion*. Blackwell: Oxford.

Collinge and Palmer (1997) *Prion Diseases*. Oxford University Press: Oxford.

Davis R (1989) *My Journey into Alzheimer's Disease*. Tyndale: Wheaton.

Dunnett S and Richards S (1998) 'What chance neural transplantation repair?' *Wellcome News Supplement 2*. Wellcome Trust: London.

Eastman M (1994) *Old Age Abuse: A new perspective*. 2nd ed. Chapman & Hall; co-published with Age Concern England.
(Now out of print but may be available from your local library.)

Economists Advisory Group (1997) *Cost of Illness: Updated final report*. Economists Advisory Group: London.

Evans E (1991) *It's Me, Grandma, it's Me*. Alzheimer's Society, Bridport Branch: Bridport.

Feil N (1982) *Validation – The Feil Method: How to help the disorientated old-old*. Edward Feil: Cleveland Ohio.

Gauthier S (1996) *Clinical Diagnosis and Management of Alzheimer's Disease*. Martin Dunitz: London.

Gray A and Fenner P (1993) 'Alzheimer's disease: the burden of the illness in England'. *Health Trends*, 25(1), pages 31-37.

Harvey RJ (1998) *Young-onset Dementia*. Imperial College School of Medicine: London.

Heywood B (1994) *Caring for Maria*. Element: Shaftesbury, Dorset.

Holland A (1993) *Down's Syndrome and Dementia*. Stirling Dementia Services Development Centre: Stirling.

Killick J (1997a) 'Communication: a matter of life and death of the mind'. *Journal of Dementia Care*, 5 (5), September 1997.

Killick J (1997b) 'You are words'. *Journal of Dementia Care*, January 1997.

Kitwood T (1995) 'Cultures of care: tradition and change'. In: Kitwood and Benson (eds) *The New Culture of Dementia Care*. Hawker: London.

Lishman WA (1994) 'History of dementia research'. In: Huppert et al (eds) *Dementia and Normal Ageing*, pages 41–56. CUP: Cambridge.

Launer LJ et al (1999) 'Regional differences in the incidence of dementia in Europe'. In: Iqbal et al (eds) *Alzheimer's disease and related disorders: etiology, pathogenesis and therapeutics*. Wiley: Chichester.

Lovestone S (1998) *Early Diagnosis and Treatment of Alzheimer's Disease*. Martin Dunitz: London.

Moniz-Cook E and Gill A (1996) 'The deep roots of folklore and superstition'. *Journal of Dementia Care*, March 1996.

Neal D (1996) 'All things bright and beautiful'. *Journal of Dementia Care*, January 1996.

Sacks O (1985) *The Man who Mistook his Wife for a Hat*. Picador: London.

Smith, AD (1998) 'Towards therapy and prevention'. *Wellcome News Supplement*. Wellcome Trust: London.

Woods R and Lay C (1996) *Caring for the Person with Dementia*. 4th ed. Alzheimer's Society: London.

Useful addresses

Action on Elder Abuse
Astral House
1268 London Road
London SW16 4ER
Tel: 020 8764 7648
Email: aea@ace.org.uk
Elder Abuse Response Line: 0808 808 8141 (10am-4.30pm weekdays)
Aims to prevent abuse of older people by raising awareness, education, promoting research and the collection and dissemination of information. Operates a confidential helpline service providing information for anyone and emotional support for those involved.

Age Exchange
The Reminiscence Centre
11 Blackheath Village
London SE3 9LA
Tel: 020 8318 9105
Fax: 020 8318 0060
Email: age-exchange@lewisham.gov.uk
Website: www.age-exchange.org.uk
Information and resources about reminiscence.

Alzheimer's Society
10 Greencoat Place
London SW1P 1PH
Tel: 020 7306 0606
Fax: 020 7306 0808
Helpline: 0845 300 0336 (local call rates)
Freephone information: 0800 027 2627
Email: Info@alzheimers.org.uk
Website: www.alzheimers.org.uk
Information, support and advice about caring for someone with Alzheimer's disease. Publishes a wide range of information sheets and other publications. Can also direct you to regional and local groups in England, Wales and Northern Ireland.

Alzheimer Scotland – Action on Dementia
22 Drumsheugh Gardens
Edinburgh EH3 7RN
Tel: 0131 243 1453
Fax: 0131 243 1450
Dementia helpline: 0808 808 3000 (24 hour)
Email: alzheimer@alzscot.org
Website: www.alzscot.org

Information and support for people with dementia and their carers in Scotland. Supports a network of carers support groups.

Alzheimer Society of Ireland
43 Northumberland Avenue
DunLaoghaire
Dublin
Tel: 00 353 1 284 6616
Fax: 00 353 1 284 6030
Email: alzheim@iol.ie
Website: www.alzheimer.ie

Information and support for people with dementia and their carers in the Republic of Ireland.

Alzheimer Europe
145 Route de Thionville
L-2611 Luxembourg
Tel: 00 352 29 79 70
Fax: 00 352 29 79 72
Email: info@alzheimer-europe.org
Website: www.alzheimer-europe.org

Aims to improve the care and treatment of people with dementia in more than 20 countries.

Alzheimer's Disease International
45-46 Lower Marsh
London SE1 7RG
Tel: 020 7620 3011
Fax: 020 7401 7351
Email: info@alz.co.uk
Website: www.alz.co.uk

An umbrella organisation of over 40 national organisations around the world.

Bradford Dementia Research Group

School of Health Studies
University of Bradford
West Yorkshire BD5 0BB
Tel: 01274 233996/236454
Fax: 01274 236395

Provides information about dementia care mapping.

Care for the Carers

Heffle Court Annexe
Station Road
Heathfield
East Sussex TN21 8DR
Tel: 01435 862376

A local organisation in East Sussex which can provide information about the Care Passport scheme.

Carers National Association

20-25 Glasshouse Yard
London EC1A 4JT
Tel: 020 7490 8818
Fax: 020 7490 8824
Carersline: 0808 808 7777

Provides information and advice if you are looking after someone, whether in your own home or at a distance. Can put you in touch with other carers and carers' groups in your area.

Carers National Association in Wales

River House
Ynysbridge Court
Gwaelod y Garth
Cardiff CF15 9SS
Tel: 029 2081 1370

Counsel and Care
Twyman House
16 Bonny Street
London NW1 9PG
Tel: 020 7485 1550
Fax: 020 7267 6877
Advice line: 0845 300 7585 (10.30am-4pm)
Email: counsel&care@counselandcare.demon.co.uk

A national advice and information service for older people on funding for residential care. Produces a range of factsheets.

Crossroads Care Attendant Scheme
10 Regent Place
Rugby
Warwickshire CV21 2PN
Tel: 01788 573653

Dementia Relief Trust
6 Camden High Street
London NW1 0JH
Tel: 020 7333 8115
Fax: 020 7333 0660
Email: dementia.relief@ukonline.co.uk
The Trust funds the Admiral Nurse schemes in six areas of London and one in Kent.

Dementia Services Development Centres (DSDC)
See page 125

Journal of Dementia Care
Hawker Publications
13 Park House
140 Battersea Park Road
London SW11 4NB
Tel: 020 7720 2108
Fax: 020 7498 3023
Email: jdc@hawkerpubs.demon.co.uk

Bi-monthly publication for professionals working in dementia care.

Public Trust Office

Stewart House
24 Kingsway
London WC2B 6JX
Tel: 020 7664 7300
Fax: 020 7664 7702

For information about taking over the affairs of someone who is mentally incapable in England or Wales. In Northern Ireland enquiries should be addressed to: The Office of Care and Protection, Royal Courts of Justice, PO Box 410, Chichester Street, Belfast BT1 3JF.

Speechmark Publishing

Telford Road
Bicester
Oxon OX6 0TS
Tel: 01869 244644
Fax: 01869 320040
Email: info@speechmark.net
Website: www.speechmark.net

Produces a range of resources suitable for use with people with dementia. (Formerly called Winslow Press.)

Dementia Services Development Centres (DSDC)

The service development centres aim to promote research and development, give training and provide information mainly for professionals working in dementia care.

Dementia North

Wolfson Research Centre
Newcastle General Hospital
Westgate Road
Newcastle Upon Tyne NE6 4BE
Tel: 0191 256 3318
Information: 0191 256 3320

Dementia Voice
Blackberry Hill Hospital
Fishponds
Bristol BS16 2EW
Tel: 0117 975 4863
Fax: 0117 965 6061
Email: office@dementia-voice.org.uk
Website: www.dementia-voice.org.uk
The DSDC for the South West of England.

London Centre for Dementia Care
Department of Psychiatry & Behavioural Sciences
University College
Wolfson Building
48 Riding House Street
London W1N 8AA
Tel: 020 7504 9475
Fax: 020 7323 1459
Email: m.orrell@ucl.ac.uk

Midlands DSDC
c/o Social Services Department
Civic Centre
St Peter's Square
Wolverhampton WV1 1RT
Tel: 01902 555306
Fax: 01902 555361

North Wales DSDC
North Wales Institute of Medicine & Social Care Research
University of Wales
Bangor
Gwynedd LL57 2UW
Tel: 01248 383719
Fax: 01248 382229
Email: dsdc@bangor.ac.uk

North West DSDC
Dover Street Building
University of Manchester
Oxford Road
Manchester M13 9PL
Tel: 0161 275 2000
Fax: 0161 275 3924
Email: amanda.bryant@man.ac.uk

Republic of Ireland Dementia Services Information and Development Centre
St James Hospital
James' Street
Dublin 8
Eire
Tel: 00 353 1 453 7941
Fax: 00 353 1 454 1796
Email: director@stjames.ie

South East DSDC
c/o Invicta Community Care NHS Trust
Priority House
Hermitage Lane
Maidstone ME16 9PH
Tel: 01622 725000 ext 290
Fax: 01622 725290
Email: equalinvicta@hotmail.com

South Wales DSDC
Service Development Team (EMI)
Royal Hamadryad Hospital
Hamadryad Road Docks
Cardiff CF10 5UQ
Tel: 029 2049 4952
Fax: 029 2049 6431
Email: sdteam@cdffcom-tr.wales.nhs.uk

Stirling DSDC
University of Stirling
Stirling FK9 4LA
Tel: 01786 467740
Fax: 01786 466846
Website: www.stir.ac.uk/dsdc

Produces a self-study pack on dementia and runs training courses in Scotland.

About Age Concern

Introducing Dementia: The essential facts and issues of care is one of a wide range of publications produced by Age Concern England, the National Council on Ageing. Age Concern works on behalf of all older people and believes later life should be fulfilling and enjoyable. For too many this is impossible. As the leading charitable movement in the UK concerned with ageing and older people, Age Concern finds effective ways to change that situation.

Where possible, we enable older people to solve problems themselves, providing as much or as little support as they need. A network of local Age Concerns, supported by 250,000 volunteers, provides community-based services such as lunch clubs, day centres and home visiting.

Nationally, we take a lead role in campaigning, parliamentary work, policy analysis, research, specialist information and advice provision, and publishing. Innovative programmes promote healthier lifestyles and provide older people with opportunities to give the experience of a lifetime back to their communities.

Age Concern is dependent on donations, covenants and legacies.

Age Concern England
1268 London Road
London SW16 4ER
Tel: 020 8765 7200
Fax: 020 8765 7211

Age Concern Scotland
113 Rose Street
Edinburgh EH2 3DT
Tel: 0131 220 3345
Fax: 0131 220 2779

Age Concern Cymru
4th Floor
1 Cathedral Road
Cardiff CF1 9SD
Tel: 029 2037 1566
Fax: 029 2039 9562

Age Concern Northern Ireland
3 Lower Crescent
Belfast BT7 1NR
Tel: 028 9024 5729
Fax: 028 9023 5497

Publications from Age Concern Books

Promoting Mobility for People with Dementia: A problem-solving approach

Rosemary Oddy

People with dementia must be enabled to move and given the opportunity to do so frequently, with or without help, if they are to remain mobile. The common sense approaches described in this book should ease the task of retaining optimum levels of mobility for people with dementia for as long as possible, without jeopardising the health and safety of those who care for them.

With the wealth of ideas contained in this book, physiotherapists, occupational therapists, nurses and carers will find plenty to stimulate the imagination.

£14.99 0-86242-242-6

Reminiscence and Recall: A guide to good practice

Faith Gibson

This revised and updated edition includes guidance on working with people with dementia, international developments and creative communications. Packed with detailed advice on planning and running successful reminiscence work, topics include:

- why reminiscence work can be valuable
- suggestions for themed topics
- using visual, audio and tactile triggers
- planning and running a reminiscence group
- inter-generational and life history work
- working with people from different cultures

This guide provides advice and support to develop and maintain the very highest standards in reminiscence work.

£11.99 0-86242-253-1

The Reminiscence Trainer's Pack

Faith Gibson

This teaching pack is designed as a straightforward teaching tool to assist trainers in presenting the basic ideas underlying planned reminiscence work. The pack aims to equip trainers in a variety of settings, sectors and service agencies primarily concerned with older people. The training is designed to introduce reminiscence workers to the theory and practice. Topics include:

- what is reminiscence?
- working with individuals and with small groups
- working with people from different cultures
- working with people with hearing, sight and speech difficulties
- working with people with dementia

£35 0-86242-305-8

If you would like to order any of these titles, please write to the address below, enclosing a cheque or money order for the appropriate amount (plus £1.95 p&p) made payable to Age Concern England. Credit card orders may be made on 0870 44 22 044 (for individuals) or 0870 44 22 120 (AC federation, other organisations and institutions).

Age Concern Books
PO Box 232
Newton Abbot
Devon TQ12 4XQ

Age Concern Information Line /Factsheets subscription

Age Concern produces 44 comprehensive factsheets designed to answer many of the questions older people (or those advising them) may have. These include factsheets about money and benefits, health, community care, leisure and education, and housing. For up to five free factsheets, telephone: 0800 00 99 66 (7am-7pm, seven days a week, every day of the year). Alternatively you may prefer to write to Age Concern, FREEPOST (SWB 30375), ASHBURTON, Devon TQ13 7ZZ.

For professionals working with older people, the factsheets are available on an annual subscription service, which includes updates throughout the year. For further details and costs of the subscription, please contact Pat Boon on 020 8765 7206, or write to her at Age Concern England's Head Office at the address on page 129.

Index